Food Quality Analysis

Food Quality Analysis

Applications of Analytical Methods Coupled With Artificial Intelligence

Edited by

ASHUTOSH KUMAR SHUKLA

Department of Physics, Ewing Christian College, Prayagraj, Uttar Pradesh, India

ELSEVIER

ACADEMIC PRESS

An imprint of Elsevier

Academic Press is an imprint of Elsevier
125 London Wall, London EC2Y 5AS, United Kingdom
525 B Street, Suite 1650, San Diego, CA 92101, United States
50 Hampshire Street, 5th Floor, Cambridge, MA 02139, United States
The Boulevard, Langford Lane, Kidlington, Oxford OX5 1GB, United Kingdom

ISBN: 978-0-323-95988-9

For Information on all Academic Press publications
visit our website at https://www.elsevier.com/books-and-journals

Publisher: Nikki P. Levy
Acquisitions Editor: Nina Bandeira
Editorial Project Manager: Andrea R. Dulberger
Production Project Manager: R. Vijay Bharath
Cover Designer: Vicky Pearson Esser

Typeset by MPS Limited, Chennai, India

Contents

List of contributors

Sumaiya Fatima
Department of Food Technology, Harcourt Butler Technical University, Kanpur, Uttar Pradesh, India

Alessandra Maia Freire
Laboratory of Nanobiotechnology (LNANO), Embrapa Genetic Resources and Biotechnology, Brasilia, Distrito Federal, Brazil; University of Brasilia (UnB), Brasilia, Distrito Federal, Brazil

Gunawan Indrayanto
Faculty of Pharmacy, Surabaya University, Surabaya, Indonesia

Vivek Kumar
Department of Food Technology, Harcourt Butler Technical University, Kanpur, Uttar Pradesh, India

Gabriella Magarelli
Laboratory of Nanobiotechnology (LNANO), Embrapa Genetic Resources and Biotechnology, Brasilia, Distrito Federal, Brazil; Laboratory of Food Safety (LSA), Embrapa Genetic Resources and Biotechnology, Brasilia, Distrito Federal, Brazil

Monalisa Mishra
Neural Developmental Biology Lab, Department of Life Science, NIT Rourkela, Rourkela, India

Seekha Naik
Neural Developmental Biology Lab, Department of Life Science, NIT Rourkela, Rourkela, India

Nithiya Rattanapanone
Department of Food Science and Technology, Faculty of Agro-Industry, Chiang Mai University, Chiang Mai, Thailand

Abdul Rohman
Faculty of Pharmacy, Gadjah Mada University, Jogyakarta, Indonesia; Center of Excellence, Institute for Halal Industry and System (IHIS), Gadjah Mada University, Yogyakarta, Indonesia; Department of Pharmaceutical Chemistry, Faculty of Pharmacy, Gadjah Mada University, Yogyakarta, Indonesia

Luciano Paulino Silva
Laboratory of Nanobiotechnology (LNANO), Embrapa Genetic Resources and Biotechnology, Brasilia, Distrito Federal, Brazil; University of Brasilia (UnB), Brasilia, Distrito Federal, Brazil

Arunima Singh
Department of Food Technology, Harcourt Butler Technical University, Kanpur, Uttar Pradesh, India

Deepika Umrao
Department of Food Technology, Harcourt Butler Technical University, Kanpur, Uttar Pradesh, India

Prinya Wongsa
Food Science and Technology Program, School of Agro-Industry, Mae Fah Luang University, Chiang Rai, Thailand

Preface

This volume intends to describe the quality analysis methods for food items coupled with artificial intelligence. This primarily covers analytical methods including spectroscopic techniques and chromatographic methods. The volume begins with an introductory chapter elaborating on the importance of food quality analysis and discusses the different approaches for compositional and chemical analysis. This chapter also highlights the importance of food quality analysis in particular reference to pandemic times. Spectroscopic techniques including Fourier transform infrared, fluorescence, and Raman spectroscopy have been covered in the following chapters. Multivariate analysis and applications of different sophisticated statistical tools have been included in these chapters in addition to the basic principles involved. A wide range of food items have been covered, which include fats and oils, beer, and other pharmaceutical materials. Electrochemical sensor applications coupled with machine learning has been discussed in a separate chapter. Interdisciplinary approach has come in a natural way as per the expertise of the contributors ranging over different disciplines.

I sincerely thank the reviewers for their valuable contribution in shaping the volume at the initial stages of proposal submission. I am especially thankful to the expert contributors for their unique contribution to this collection. I am also thankful to Nina Bandeira, Food Science Acquisitions Editor, Elsevier, for giving me the opportunity to present this book to the readers. My thanks are also due to Andrea Dulberger, Editorial Project Manager, Elsevier, for her support during different stages of the project.

June 2022

Ashutosh Kumar Shukla

CHAPTER ONE

Importance of food quality analysis in relation to food safety and human health and COVID-19 in particular

Vivek Kumar, Deepika Umrao and Sumaiya Fatima
Department of Food Technology, Harcourt Butler Technical University, Kanpur, Uttar Pradesh, India

1.1 Introduction

Population growth is directly proportional to the food market growth because it is a game of demand and supply. The food market indulges all different varieties of fresh and processed food items. Accordingly, it is divided into different segments: meat, fish, seafood, vegetables, fruits, dairy and egg products, bakery and other cereal products, spreads, sweeteners, snacks, sauces and pet food. Statistical data has shown that the food market revenue is about US$8,773,679 million in 2022 and is expected to increase by 4.79% annually till 2027. Moreover, an average volume per person in the food market is estimated to be 337.8 kg in 2022 [1]. The mentioned data clearly depicts the increasing market size of the food industry. The strict monitoring and quality analysis of food products by following quality management system play very important role in maintaining health benefits and safety of the food product as well as consistent growth of the food industry. This can be achieved by regular practice and concern of all involved in food production, processing, quality control, transportation, and storage. Moreover, if a food company sells a dangerous or poisonous product, it would be commercially devastating as well as unappealing to customers. A food may be deemed dangerous if it includes harmful bacteria (e.g., *Listeria*, *Salmonella*), poisonous chemicals (e.g., pesticides, herbicides), or foreign debris (e.g., glass, metal). As a result, it is critical that food makers adopt all possible measures to guarantee that these dangerous components are not present

Food Quality Analysis.
DOI: https://doi.org/10.1016/B978-0-323-95988-9.00003-5

or are successfully removed before the food is ingested. This can be accomplished by adhering to the government's good manufacturing practice rules for specific food items, as well as having analytical procedures capable of detecting dangerous compounds [2]. In many cases, it is critical to apply analytical procedures with high sensitivity, that is, those that can consistently identify minute amounts of harmful material. Food producers and government laboratories frequently examine food items to ensure that they are free of dangerous contaminants and that the food manufacturing facility is running properly.

As discussed, food safety is primarily important, for both manufacturers and the consumer, and thus, compositional and chemical analyses of food are very important. Complete knowledge of the food composition is essential to predict its impact on human health. The qualitative analysis of major food components like water, fat, proteins, carbohydrates, vitamins, and minerals is necessarily done owing to their nutritional importance, desirable functional properties and their effect on food safety [3]. In contrast to the macronutrients, the presence of food allergens and adulterants, even in a minute amount, is undesirable, therefore food products are also tested for their presence. Also, the food producers are always attempting to expand their market share and earnings in a highly competitive business. To achieve this, they must guarantee that their products are of greater quality, less priced, and more appealing than their competitors, while also being safe and healthy. To satisfy these stringent criteria, food makers must use analytical techniques to examine food components before, during, and after the production process to guarantee that the finished product satisfies the appropriate standards [4]. Also, in the recent years, consumer preferences have significantly shifted to healthier, higher-quality, lower-cost, and more exotic meals, and to remain competitive in the food sector, individual food makers must adapt quickly to these developments. To address these expectations, food producers frequently employ a team of scientists whose major goal is to conduct research that will result in the invention of new goods, the enhancement of current ones, and the decrease of production costs. This also requires use of analytical techniques to specify the food properties (texture, color, flavor, etc.) and to determine the role of each food component in overall properties of foods [5].

Clearly, food analysis is a branch of analytical chemistry essential to provide information on chemical composition, food processing, the presence of contaminants in food, nutritional labeling, and food quality control. Also, analysis of food products is a prerequisite to ascertain implementation of regulatory enforcements and to keep a check on compliance with national and international food laws. Among the various parameters, compositional and chemical analyses of foods are very crucial in terms of food safety and human health. Additionally, with the emergence of COVID-19, the analysis of virus-contaminated food and their ill health effects have also emerged as a major concern in food analysis. Hence, in this chapter, various food analysis techniques for different parameters are discussed under the light of their impact on food safety and human health.

1.2 Importance of food quality analysis

Nowadays, customers are well-educated and concerned about their eating habits, and they want to know the nutritional statistics listed on product labels during the purchase of packaged foods. Furthermore, testing of food items for numerous allergens contained in cereals, pulses and animal meals, pesticides and fertilizer residues, genetically modified food products, etc. is crucial for maintaining food safety. Today's population is concerned with understanding diet–health linkages, which makes it difficult for the food business to manufacture goods with balanced nutritional values and low- or zero-fat content. Food nutritional value preservation is important for food scientists as it is connected to human health, such as the association between cancer and dietary fat, cholesterol and heart disease, dietary carbohydrate and diabetes, and so on. Consequently, requirements of analytical methods are essential to justify these claims [6].

Besides, the market size of the food products is huge competition-driven, and therefore, food companies have to produce best-quality food products that meet the consumers demands. Analytical techniques play a major role in the whole food supply chain initially from the raw material to the final product quality. In the present generation of technology, manufacturers depend on the specific suppliers to perform the compositional analysis with detailed ingredient proportion as well as physiochemical and microbial characteristics. In addition, these specific analyses are depicted as a certificate of analysis with the raw material or ingredients. Another scenario is related to the maximum retail price of the final product, which also solely depends on the techniques used in the whole process to develop a certain food product. For instance, in the dairy field business, the presence of butterfat composition in bulk tanks determines the amount of money that milk producers get from the consumer, just like the amount of protein content in the flour decides the flour price and derived products' value. These are some specific products' examples that suggest an essential requirement of analytical techniques in food science to ensure the quality and reliability of the food products [7].

Also, to provide safe, healthy, and high-quality products in the national and international market, food manufacturing companies have directed their attention toward government guidelines and policies related to specific food product categories that also fulfill the standards of international rules and regulations. Food scientists must understand and be aware of these guidelines, policies, and regulations during food quality analysis. Different standard terminology and understanding have to be taken under consideration to provide best-quality food products. According to international rules and regulation, food analysis indulges nutrition labeling regulations, good manufacturing practice (GMP), Hazard Analysis Critical Control Point protocols highly in demand by food companies during establishing firms and customers [8]. Furthermore, another regulation known as the General Agreement on Tariffs and Trade (GATT) has been passed to strengthen the Codex by assigning them as an internationally principal standard managing group for the safety and quality of the food products [9]. In addition, the International Organization for Standardization (ISO) also plays a critical role in handling standards of quality management and performance. Its agenda is based on product specificity, customer satisfaction, and focuses on a process layout followed for quality management [10]. Other regional and country-specific organizations also published better quality food standards rules and regulations to provide knowledge relevant to food composition analysis. The role of specific organizations [7,11] to ensure the safety of processed foods is summarized in Table 1.1.

Moreover, compositional analysis of foods is required owing to its nutritional importance, desirable functional qualities, and impact on food safety. Along with the study of food components, chemical analysis of food is crucial to ensure safe food consumption. Chemical analysis of foods includes analysis of pH, enzyme, and food contaminants and is an essential feature of a quality assurance protocol in the food processing industries starting from the receiving of raw materials, during processing, and in the finished products. The chemical analysis feature is also essential in formulating innovative products, evaluation of processes for building food products, and identification of problems present with the unacceptable food attributes. Different parameters must be considered while forming a consumer-derived food product. Food-related health issues can be avoided by asking some questions as shown in Fig. 1.1 that

Table 1.1 List of common food safety standard organizations and their roles.

Food safety standards organizations	Roles
Saudi Arabian Standards organization	Publishing standard protocols regarding documents (labeling, testing methods)
European Commission	Stating standards for food additives
Food and Drug Administration	Protection and promotion of public health through the control and supervision of food safety
Federal Ministry of Food and Agriculture	Provides publications to promote a balanced and healthy diet
United States department of Agriculture	responsible for development and execution of federal laws food
Food Chemicals Codex	Characterization and purity of food additives, chemicals
Food Standards Agency	Protects public health by ensuring food safety
World Health Organization (WHO) expert Committee on Food Additives	Purity for food additives
Ministry of Food and Drug Safety	Promotion of public health by ensuring the food safety
Indonesian Food and Drug Authority	Protects public health through control and supervision of food safety
New Zealand Food Safety	Responsible for food safety, controls import and export of food products
Food Safety and Standards Authority of India.	Action regarding food safety and regulation in India

can be answer-responsive by analyzing different types of samples in a food processing system [12].

After completing the selection and preparation of food samples, the assay methods specific for each component present in the specific sample are performed. At the end of each analysis technique, process scientists or food analysts must perform the interpretation of the results, by making precise calculation to interpret the data in a correct manner. Data interpretation plays an important role in measuring central tendency, source of errors, specificity, sensitivity, limit of detection, precision, accuracy, and regression analysis [13]. Various methods are available in the literature to tackle food quality analysis issues that have proven specific to the food product compositions. To develop innovative methods for analysis, food analysts must understand the different criteria shown in Fig. 1.2, for production of good-quality food products following all quality analysis protocols [7].

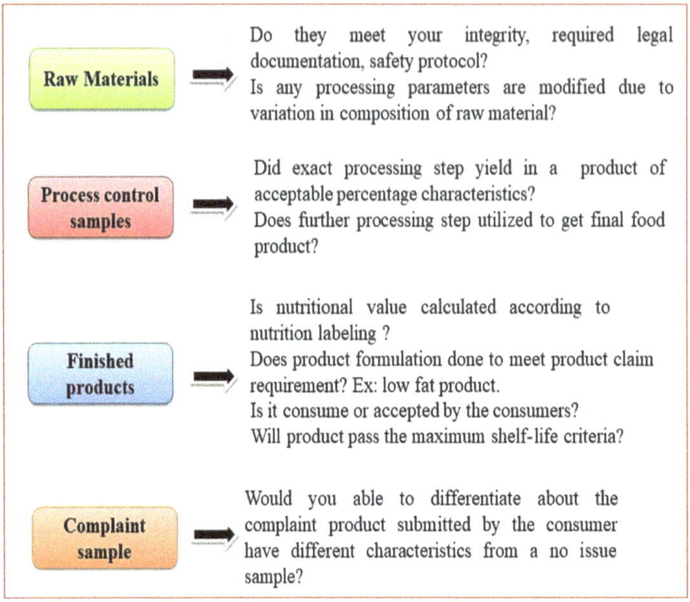

Figure 1.1 Sample analysis scheme according to food product quality assurance program.

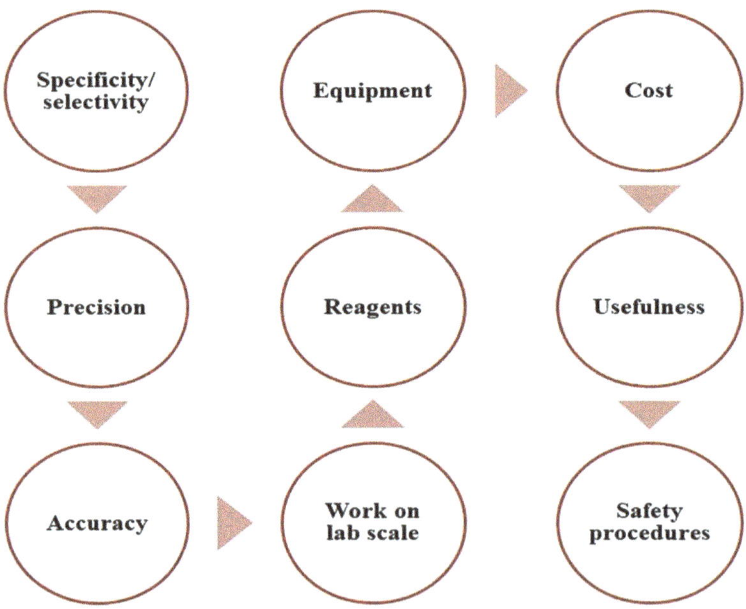

Figure 1.2 Protocol for selection of food analysis methods.

1.3 Compositional analysis of foods

Compositional analysis of foods includes the analysis of macro- and microcomponents of food, namely, moisture, fat, protein, carbohydrate, vitamins, and minerals. Each component is nutritionally significant and plays a critical role in the delegation of distinct functional qualities to diverse food items, and thus, compositional analysis of food is very critical to estimate food safety. Also, food compositional analysis has been applied to ascertain the nutritional importance of the target food component to facilitate international and national organizations for the development and implementation of effective intervention programs to enhance development of nutritionally balanced food product. Another significant reason to analyze food composition is to estimate the nutrient intake from individual food products. The data gathered from compositional analysis can be utilized for displaying dietary guidelines containing essential information on specific food attributes that are responsible for different nutritional factors required by humans and animals. Furthermore, compositional analysis gives authenticated details and facts about chemical nature of nutrients and their interaction with other biomolecules and thus provides information about the nutrient bioavailability characteristics. Nowadays, food scientists are working toward analysis of nonnutritive food components, by considering the critical role of biologically active secondary metabolites derived from plant cells (polyphenols/carotenoids). Another side of ascertaining food composition is to examine contaminants that can negatively affect consumers' health. For instance, the food chain is polluted with different classified agrochemicals, industrially produced pollutants/substances formed in place of food processing industry [14]. Therefore, a significant risk assessment protocol is required to work on data on exposure and presence of contaminants in foods. In today's era, increasing population relying on community nutritional facts, catering, concern about heathy menu cards can incline consumers' diets and significantly contribute toward nutrient supply. The formulation and implementation of standard and specific guidelines also require food composition databases to form healthy meals. The following section includes the significance of various compositional analysis techniques for different food products, as well as to highlight the impact of food components on food safety and human health.

1.3.1 Moisture analysis

Moisture content of food is one of the most important quality parameters and has economic importance to both producer and consumer. It has great significance for texture, taste, shelf-life, ease of processing, and cost of the food products. The moisture content of many processed foods such as snacks, dried foods, fried foods, baked foods, etc. greatly affect their texture and taste. Grains of high moisture content are highly susceptible to mold growth. The moisture content has direct correlation with microbial growth and therefore directly influences the shelf-life of the food products because increase in water activity in a food sample raises its susceptibility to microbial growth, which results in damage to food products and decreases their shelf-life. The rate of oxidation and browning reaction in fried foods and dehydrated fruits and vegetables increases with increase of moisture content. The optimum moisture content of raw materials is also required for ease of processing and to get the right-quality final products. The amount of moisture content can affect the physical and chemical properties of food, which are directly correlated to the freshness, pliability, and stability of food products during storage. Fig. 1.3 describes the important instances in which moisture analysis is essential to the food maker [15].

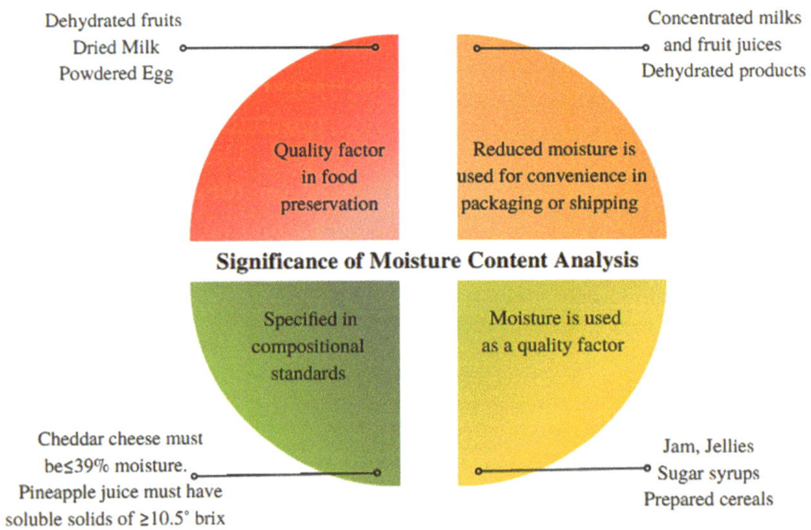

Figure 1.3 Significance of moisture content analysis.

Keeping all aspects in the mind, analysis of total moisture content in food products is essential for maintaining their quality and ensuring their safety till consumption. Moisture assays are the most difficult processes from which to avail accurate and precise facts and data [12]. Various techniques for moisture analysis with their principles, procedures, and applications are presented in Table 1.2. The most popular techniques for estimation of moisture content include oven-drying method, chemical methods, and physical methods [16]. In case of oven-drying method, the sample is heated under specific circumstances, and the weight loss is utilized to quantify the moisture content in the food sample. Forced-draft oven-drying and vacuum oven-drying are some commonly used oven-drying methods to determine the amount of moisture in foods. The time required to dry the sample completely is different for different food products and depends upon the amount of moisture present and geometrical arrangement of the food constituents [17]. However, in case of chemical method, Karl Fischer titration method comes into picture and is most suited for low-moisture-containing food commodities like candies, chocolates, dried fruits, vegetables, etc. [18]. Also, physical methods including assessment of dielectric properties, hydrometry, refractometry, and infrared analysis are also utilized to calculate the amount of moisture content in various food matrices [19–21].

1.3.2 Fat analysis

The fat content of foods is an important parameter for both consumers and food industry professionals. Lipids including fats are one of the main constituents of food and are important in our diets for a variety of reasons. They are the major source of energy, act as carrier of fat-soluble vitamins, are important constituent of cell membrane, and provide essential lipid nutrients. However, excessive consumption of some lipid components, namely, saturated fat, trans fat, and cholesterol are harmful for human health [22]. Saturated and trans fats are responsible for high risk of coronary artery disease and cardiovascular diseases [23]. Furthermore, elevated levels of LDL (low-density lipoprotein), commonly called "bad cholesterol," increases heart diseases. In order to limit the detrimental effects of lipid constituents on human health, WHO has issued recommendations for dietary fat intake. Recommended levels of total, saturated, and trans fat expressed as percent of energy are 20%–25%, $<$10%, and $<$1%, respectively [24]. Apart from biological importance, the lipid component plays an important role in establishing the physical characteristics of food, such as texture, flavor, mouthfeel, and appearance. Hence, development

Table 1.2 Techniques used for analysis of moisture content in foods.

S. NO	Name of technique	Operating principle	Application	Reference
1	Forced draft oven-drying	Food products are heated under specific condition and determine the loss of weight to analyze moisture content	Butter milk, cheese, chocolate, cocoa, egg albumin, ice cream	[17]
2	Karl Fischer titration	Titration technique based on the oxidation reaction between Sulfur dioxide and iodine	Applied in low-moisture-content foods; dried fruits and vegetables, candies, coffee, oils	[18]
3	Dielectric method	Determining the change in resistance or capacitance to an electric current passed through a food samples	Limited to food samples has moisture content range 30%–35%; cereal grains	[19]
4	Hydrometry	Measurement of specific gravity with hydrometer or pycnometer	Beverages, salt brines, sugar solutions, and solids composition in milk	[19]
5	Refractometry	Unknown chemical compound in the sample has specific refractive index, thus it is utilized in measurement of its qualitative identification by comparing its RI value with reported values	Moisture content in liquid sugar and condensed milk	[20]
6	Infrared analysis	Works on absorption of radiation by chemical molecules present in foods	Utilized in milk analyzer to detect fat, lactose, protein, and total solids in milk	[21]

of low-fat alternatives to many foods is difficult, owing to undesirable effects on physical and functional properties of food [25,26]. However, many fats are prone to oxidation, which leads to the formation of potentially harmful free radicals and off-flavor in the food products. Thus, qualitative and quantitative analysis of fats is an important aspect of food safety and food quality, along with its significance in accurate nutritional labeling on packaged foods and certainty in meeting manufacturer's specifications for desirable functional properties of food (Fig. 1.4).

Fats are nonpolar compounds soluble in organic solvents and insoluble in water. This fundamental is used as a basis for separation of fats from other food components. Fats have a range of relative hydrophobicity, and hence, the extraction solvent is selected on the basis of solubility of a particular fat, for example, glycolipids are soluble in alcohols and have low solubility in hexane, whereas triacylglycerols are most soluble in hexane. The major fat properties analyzed by food analysts are total fat concentration, physicochemical properties of fat, and composition of fat in food matrix. However, from health and food safety point of view, determination of total lipid/fat content is most important. The analytical techniques to quantify fat content in different foods have been categorized as solvent extraction methods, nonsolvent extraction methods, and instrumental methods [27] (Table 1.3). Solvent extraction method for fat estimation is performed as a batch, semicontinuous, and continuous processes [28,29]. Sample preparation and selection of appropriate solvent are vital for accurate results and depend on the food matrix being analyzed. The fat content of almost all types of food matrices except the liquid foods like milk can be determined by these methods. For milk and milk products, nonsolvent wet extraction methods are generally used. These methods are based

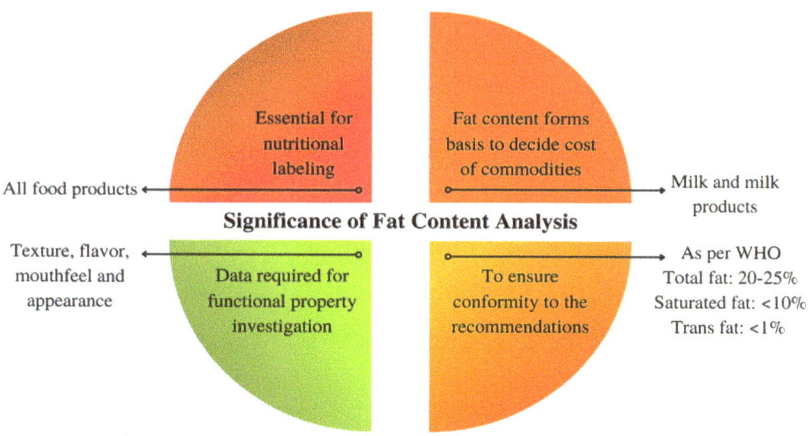

Figure 1.4 Significance of fat content analysis.

Table 1.3 Techniques used for analysis of total fat content in foods.

Name of technique	Operating principle	Application	Reference
Solvent extraction methods			
Batch solvent extraction	Method based on mixing organic solvent and sample vigorously and allowing it to separate into two phases. The liquid phase is decanted, and solvent is evaporated leaving behind the lipid	Cereal, meat, baked goods, etc.	[28]
Semicontinuous solvent Extraction (Soxhlet method)	Technique based on solvent build up in extraction chamber for 5–10 min, where it surrounds the sample completely and then elicits back to boiling flask. The fat content is determined by the loss in weight of the sample		[29]
Continuous solvent extraction (goldfish method)	Method based on continuous flow of solvent from boiling flask over the sample held in ceramic filter. The fat content is determined by the loss in weight of the sample		[16]
Nonsolvent wet extraction methods			
Babcock method	Technique based on addition of sulfuric acid in milk sample, which digests protein and releases fat. The mixture is then centrifuged for isolation and quantification of fat	Milk and its products except sugar- and chocolate-containing products	[30]

(*Continued*)

Table 1.3 (Continued)

Name of technique	Operating principle	Application	Reference
Gerber method	Technique used in this method is same as Babcock method, except the use of amyl alcohol	Milk and its products	[30]
Instrumental methods			
Infrared method	Method based on absorption of infrared energy by fat molecules at 5.73 μm. The higher the amount of energy absorbed, the higher would be the fat content of the sample	Meats, cereals, and oilseeds	[31]
Specific gravity (Foss-Let method)	Based on specific gravity of sample solvent extract, extricated with perchloroethylene	Meat and meat products	[32]
Nuclear Magnetic resonance	Technique can be used to determine fatty acid profile, solid fat content, and to monitor oxidation of fats	Edible oils and fats	[33]

on extraction of milk fat by concentrated sulfuric acid followed by its isolation and quantification. Babcock and Gerber methods are the commonly used wet extraction methods for estimation of fat in milk and its products [30]. Apart from the aforementioned methods, certain instrumental methods can also be employed for fat analysis in food samples. Infrared method, based on absorption of infrared energy by fat at 5.73 nm wavelength, is used to estimate fat content in cereals, meat, and oil seeds [31]. On the other hand, application of specific gravity (Foss-Let) method for meat and meat products has been reported [32]. Additionally, nuclear magnetic resonance techniques can be used to highlight the fat profiles in various food matrices and therefore have wide application in detection of adulterant in edible oil, along with it being an affordable and non-destructive tool for measuring the total fat content [33].

1.3.3 Protein analysis

Proteins are the polymers of amino acids. They are the body-building foods, which, along with carbohydrates and fats, act as a source of energy. They contain essential amino acids responsible for numerous physiological functions in the human body. Also, proteins perform various biological functions, for instance, they act as enzyme catalysts, are structural components of food and responsible for its texture (in meat and fish products), responsible for transportation of essentials in the human body (e.g., transportation of oxygen done by hemoglobin), act as storage proteins (egg albumen, seed proteins), and show antibiotic nature (immunoglobins). Besides, proteins provide unique functional properties to foods [34]. Typically, proteins are used as emulsifiers, stabilizers, gelling agents, foaming agents, and thickeners. Talking about human health and food safety menaces associated with proteins, they pose adverse health effects only when consumed above recommended dietary allowances. Disorder of bone and calcium homeostasis, liver and renal functions, along with increased cancer risk and precipitated progression of coronary artery diseases are the few detrimental health effects associated with high intake of proteins over a long period of time [35]. Also, the presence of allergens, which are proteinaceous in nature, also causes deleterious consequences in sensitive individuals. In addition to the effect of protein on human health, they can affect the stability and shelf-life of foods by enhancing antioxidant activity, imparting antimicrobial activity (nisin: antibacterial peptide used to preserve cheese, meat, and fish), and affecting the gas permeability in edible coating and bio-packaging material [36]. Therefore, the analysis of protein content in foods is essential from human health and food safety perspective. Moreover, protein analysis is essential for nutritional labeling, pricing, functional property investigation, and biological activity determination [37] (Fig. 1.5).

Analysis of protein content in foods is complicated as other major food components, namely, lipids and carbohydrates, interfere with the analysis. The basic principle for determination of protein content in foods includes estimation of its nitrogen content. However, nonprotein nitrogen coming from urea, uric acids, free amino acids, peptides, amino sugars, porphyrins, etc. possibly affect the estimated value. Hence, a correction factor is introduced. The correction factor is nitrogen-to-protein conversion factor, which is different for different foods owing to their amino acid profile. In addition to estimation of nitrogen content, peptide bonds, aromatic amino

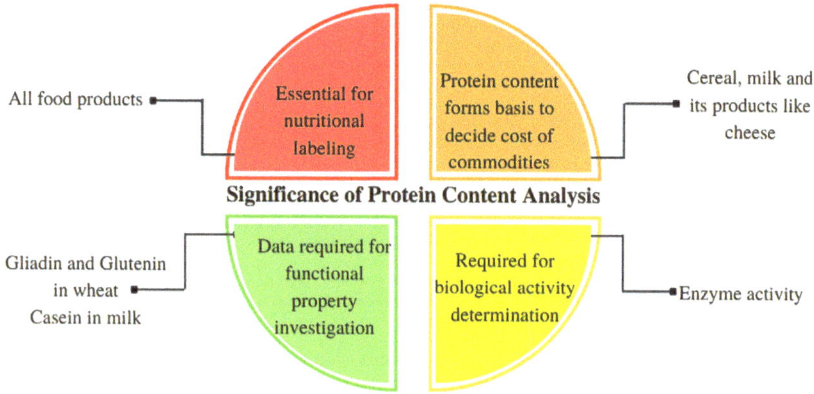

Figure 1.5 Significance of protein content analysis.

acids, ultraviolet absorptivity of proteins, dye-binding capacity, and light-scattering properties often form basis to determine protein content in various food samples [37]. The different methods adopted for protein estimation are summarized in Table 1.4. Kjeldahl method and Dumas method of protein estimation are based on amount of nitrogen content in the food matrices. The former estimates protein content by digesting the food sample followed by distillation and titration to quantify nitrogen in terms of ammonium salts and is applicable to all types of food samples [38]. Alternative to Kjeldahl method is Dumas (nitrogen combustion method), in which the food sample is combusted in presence of oxygen to convert all nitrogenous component into free nitrogen or nitrous oxide, which is subsequently quantified [39]. Both these methods require conversion of % nitrogen into % protein with appropriate conversion factor, specific to each food product. Also, the application of infrared spectroscopy has been reported for estimating protein content in milk, cereal, grains, and meat samples [40,41]. In addition to the above methods, protein content can be estimated in terms of peptide bonds as in case of Biuret method [38,39], Lowry method [42], and bicinchoninic acid method [43]. Protein estimation of milk and meat samples has also been reported by other methods including dye-binding methods [43–45] and ultraviolet absorption methods [46,47].

1.3.4 Carbohydrate analysis

Carbohydrates are the macronutrient present in food and act as a major source of energy for human body. They are found in the form of sugars,

Table 1.4 Techniques used for analysis of protein content in foods.

Name of technique	Operating principle	Application	Reference
Kjeldahl method	Technique based on digestion of food sample with sulfuric acid, which converts organic nitrogen to ammonium sulfates. The digest is then neutralized with alkali and distilled into acidic medium. The distillate is then titrated with standard alkali to calculate % protein using the conversion factor	All types of food samples	[38]
Dumas (nitrogen combustion) method	Food sample is combusted in oxygen; all nitrogenous component in it gets converted into free nitrogen and nitrous oxide, which are reduced to nitrogen in copper reduction column and finally quantified by gas chromatography using a thermal conductivity detector	Alternative to Kjeldahl method. Suitable for all types of food	[39]
Infrared spectroscopy	Works on absorption of radiation by chemical molecules present in foods	Milk samples, cereals, grains, and meat products	[40,41]
Biuret method	Method based on estimation of absorbance for resultant purple colored mixture developed due reaction between peptide bonds and cupric ions in alkaline medium	Cereals, meat, soyabean proteins	[48,49]
Lowry method	Estimates protein concentration by calculating reactivity of peptide bonds and oxidation of aromatic amino acids	All types of food samples	[42]

(*Continued*)

Table 1.4 (Continued)

Name of technique	Operating principle	Application	Reference
Dye-binding methods	Protein binds with the dye and gives a characteristic color	Milk, wheat, soy products and meat	[44,45]
Bicinchoninic acid method	Peptide bond reduces the cupric ion in alkaline reagent, which then reacts with bicinchoninic acid to give characteristic purple color	Limited to isolates and not suitable for complex food systems	[43]
Ultraviolet absorption method	Absorption of ultraviolet light at 280 nm due to presence of tryptophan and tyrosine residues in the proteins	Milk and meat products	[46,47]

starches, and fibers and serve as fuel for brain, heart muscles, and kidneys and aid digestion along with other physiological functions [50]. Fibers are non-digestible polysaccharides that promote digestive health by regulating normal bowel movement and help in lowering cholesterol levels. However, starches are broken into sugars, which are then metabolized to generate energy. The rate of digestion and absorption of carbohydrates affects the blood glucose level. Hyperglycemia (high blood sugar levels) may damage blood vessels and increase risk of heart disease, heart stroke, kidney disease, and nerves problems [51]. Along with their impact on human health, carbohydrates conduce to functional attributes like body, bulk density, viscosity, water-holding capacity, flavors, browning, stability in emulsions, and desirable textures [52]. Owing to nutritional and functional importance of carbohydrates, their quantitative analysis is essential. Carbohydrate analysis is also important to ensure conformity to government regulations on specific constituent along with its role in nutritional labeling of foods and detection of food adulteration.

Commonly, carbohydrate content of food can be estimated by conducting proximate analysis for other food components and subtracting them from unity. However, this method gives erroneous results as a consequence of experimental errors; hence, it is better to quantify carbohydrates by direct methods. Numerous analytical methods for estimation of monosaccharide, oligosaccharide, and polysaccharide have been reported in the literature (Table 1.5).

Table 1.5 Techniques used for analysis of carbohydrates content in foods.

Name of technique	Operating principle	Application	Reference
Monosaccharide and oligosaccharide analysis			
Chromatographic method	Works on separation of carbohydrates on the basis of their differential adsorption characteristics by passing its solution through an analyzing column. Chromatographic technique along with spectrometry helps in identification of chemical structure of compounds	Monosaccharides, oligosaccharides, and hydrolyzed polysaccharides	[52]
Electrophoretic methods	Separation based on electrophoretic mobility of ions under the application of voltage	Fruit juices, syrups	[53]
Chemical method	Based on determination of reducing sugar concentration in samples, quantified by gravimetric method, titration, or by colorimetric reactions	Honey, fruit juices	[54–56]
Enzymatic method	Method based on estimation of carbohydrates facilitated by observation of specific enzymes reaction	Monosaccharides, oligosaccharides, and polysaccharides in food samples	[52]
Specific gravity method	Determines concentration of carbohydrate solution by measuring specific gravity of solution and comparing with predetermined charts	Accurate only for pure sucrose and solutions of a single substance	[52]

(*Continued*)

Table 1.5 (Continued)

Name of technique	Operating principle	Application	Reference
Refractive index method	Estimates total solids in sample solution based on the change in direction of electromagnetic waves on passing from one medium to another	Juices, jam, syrups, honey, molasses, etc.	[57]
Spectroscopic method	Works on absorption of radiation by chemical molecules present in foods	Fruits, vegetables, honey, milk, etc.	[58]
Starch: Degree of gelatinization analysis			
Enzymatic method	Based on the fact that gelatinization increases the chemical reactivity of inert starch granules toward amylolytic enzymes	Maize starch	[59]
Starch: Retrogradation analysis			
Rheological method	Studies development of polymer structure by rapid visco analyser	Gels, starch, bread	[60,61]
Thermal analysis	Technique based on changes in heat flux during starch retrogradation	Potato, maize, and wheat starch	[62]
Spectroscopic method	Works on absorption of radiation by chemical molecules present in foods	Rice and wheat starch	[63,64]
Dietary fiber analysis			
Crude fiber method	Estimates indigestible fiber by sequential acid and alkali treatments of defatted food samples	Applicable for all food matrix	[65]

(Continued)

Table 1.5 (Continued)

Name of technique	Operating principle	Application	Reference
Total soluble and insoluble fiber method	Based on removal of starch and protein from food samples by enzymatic reactions, followed by recovery of soluble and insoluble fiber by alcohol treatment	Used in analysis of cereal, fruits, vegetable, and processed foods	[52]

Monosaccharides and oligosaccharides are estimated by various techniques like chromatography [52], electrophoretic methods [53], chemical methods [54–57], enzymatic methods [56], and physical methods [57,58], as discussed in Table 1.5. The starch content is mainly important from functional aspect; hence, its degree of gelatinization and retrogradation are usually determined. Enzymatic methods are employed to analyze the degree of starch gelatinization [59]; however, use of rheological methods [60,61], thermal analysis [62], and spectroscopic methods [63,64] has been reported to study retrogradation in starch. For estimation of dietary fiber content, gravimetric methods [65] and chemical methods are employed.

1.3.5 Vitamin analysis

Vitamins, also called vital amines, are nutritionally indispensable micronutrients. They are essential for various physiological activities of the body including their functions as coenzymes and precursors (thiamin, niacin, riboflavin, biotin, etc.), antioxidants (ascorbic acid and tocopherols), components involved in genetic regulation system (carotenoid and calciferol) and some specialized functions specific to each vitamin (vitamin A responsible for vision, vitamin C for hydroxylation reaction, vitamin K essential for carboxylation reactions, etc.) [66]. Consequently, their inadequate supply results in deficiency diseases, and excess intake is also undesirable. Food authorities have issued recommendations for intake levels of each vitamin. To ensure conformity to the recommendations, quantitative analysis of vitamins is essential. Moreover, analysis of vitamins plays crucial role in estimation of nutritional requirements of humans other than ensuring accurate values on food labeling [67]. In addition to the role of vitamins in human health, they influence the chemical nature of foods, establishing safety of processed foods. They act as reducing agents, reactants in browning, radical scavengers, and flavor precursors, thus adding to the necessity of quantitative analysis of vitamins.

Three types of methods are used for the analysis of vitamins, namely, bioassays, microbiological assays, and physiochemical or chemical assays [67]. Bioassay methods involve animals and humans as test organisms in its analysis. As of now, Vitamin B_{12} and D are analyzed by this method. However, microbiological assay method employs bacteria, yeast, and protozoan organisms for analysis and is limited to water-soluble vitamins [57—70]. It is based on the fact that growth of microorganisms is comparable to the presence of a specific vitamin. Physicochemical methods include fluorometric, spectrometric, chromatographic, radiometric, and enzymatic techniques, as presented in Table 1.6. High-performance liquid chromatography (HPLC) is the most widely used chromatographic techniques for estimation of both water- and fat-soluble vitamins present in milk, oil, juices, etc. [71,72]. On the other hand, spectroscopic methods are applied to determine fat-soluble vitamins in oil and milk [73], and fluorometric method, enzymatic method, and radiometric methods are reported to measure water-soluble vitamins, especially vitamin C and vitamin B in fruit juices and breakfast cereals, respectively [74—76].

1.3.6 Mineral analysis

Minerals are minor components of foods essential for maintenance of life. Both inadequate and excess intake of minerals are undesirable and can lead to disorders specific to the imbalance of particular mineral. They are classified into macro, trace, and ultra-trace minerals depending on their daily requirements in the human body. Macro minerals, namely, phosphorus, calcium, potassium, sodium, magnesium, sulfur, and chloride, are required at 100 mg/day for an adult. On the other hand, iron, zinc, iodine, copper, manganese, fluoride, chromium, selenium, silica, and molybdenum make up trace minerals that are required in milligrams per day. Tin, arsenic, vanadium, nickel, and boron are required only in trace quantities, and their possible biological functions are still being investigated. Another category of minerals exists in nature that are toxic to human health, specifically, lead, mercury, aluminum, and cadmium [77]. Even some essential minerals like fluoride and selenium when consumed in excess quantities are toxic. Thus, the levels of mineral intake need to be known/controlled, and this can be achieved with accurate analysis of minerals. Also, Nutritional Labelling and Education Act (1990) made it

Table 1.6 Physiochemical techniques used for analysis of vitamin content in foods.

Name of technique	Operating principle	Application	Reference
Bioassay methods	Based on study of pharmacological effects on animals	Vitamin A and vitamin D in liquid supplements	[68,69]
Microbiological assay methods	Based on quantification of vitamins as the growth of microorganisms is proportional to vitamin in the substrate	Limited to water-soluble vitamins	[70]
Physiochemical methods			
Chromatography method	Based on separation of components from a mixture applied on stationary phase, when it travels by the help of mobile phase	Water- and fat-soluble vitamins in milk, oils, fruit juices, etc.	[71]
Spectroscopic method	Works on absorption of radiation by chemical molecules present in foods	Fat soluble vitamins in milk and oil samples	[73]
Fluorometric method	Technique based on analysis of fluorescence produced in a sample	Vitamin C in juices	[74]
Enzymatic method	Based on colorimetric detection of products	Vitamin C in fruit and vegetables	[75]
Radiometric method	Assay based on transformation of radioactive substrate to a radioactive product	Vitamin B_6 in breakfast cereals	[76]

mandatory to display contents of iron, calcium, and sodium owing to their crucial roles in preventing anemia, obstructing osteoporosis condition, and controlling hypertension, respectively. The inclusion of other minerals on the label, however, is optional unless minerals are a part of nutritional claim of the processed foods [78]. Moreover, the increasing demands of fortified foods and effect of water hardness on different food products are some instances justifying the importance of quantitative analysis of minerals from nutritional and functional perspective.

Separation and quantification principle are applied as a basis for mineral analysis. Minerals are separated from food matrix by either specific methods such as complexometric titrations, precipitation titrations or nonspecific methods like acid extraction, ashing, etc. [78]. In specific separation method, the measurements are based on nonspecific procedures, for instance the volume of titrant is correlated with the mass of mineral [79,80], whereas, nonspecific separation techniques employed specific measurement procedures such as ion selective electrodes, colorimetry, atomic absorption spectroscopy, etc. [81–83]. Furthermore, sample preparation is required, which is unique for conforming estimation method. The various methods for quantitative analysis of minerals are summarized in Table 1.7.

Table 1.7 Techniques used for analysis of mineral content in foods.

Name of technique	Operating principle	Application	Reference
Complexometric titration	Based on volumetric titration, whose end point is indicated by the formation of a colored complex	Calcium and magnesium in water	[79]
Precipitation titration	Titration technique involves formation of a precipitate	Well suited for high-chloride foods such as cheese, meat, savories, etc.	[80]
Colorimetric methods	Consists of chromogen, which reacts with specific mineral to produce color, which is quantified by the help of absorbance values	Applicable to wide range of food matrices, including meat and its products	[81]
Ion-selective electrodes	Based on ion-selective sensors, employed to detect specific cations and anions	Processed meat, cheese, milk, wine, butter, soft drinks, etc.	[82]
Atomic absorbance spectroscopy	Works on aspiration, aerosolization, and combustion of liquified sample, which facilitates release of specific atoms that can be detected	Meat, fish, dairy products, fruit juices, etc.	[83]

1.4 Chemical analysis of foods

Chemical analysis of food refers to the study of chemical composition and structure of foods, performed to ensure safe consumption, integrity, and quality of food products. Chemical analysis, together with compositional analysis, provides critical information for determination of food properties to establish supply of desirable food products. Moreover, chemical analysis of food samples acts as prerequisite for corroborating correct nutritional information on the processed food packets and protecting the consumers against misbranded foods [84]. Apart from its essential role in nutritional labeling, chemical analysis promotes testing of food authenticity, inspection, and grading. Also, food industry being highly competitive, food manufacturers must produce economic and higher-quality food products in order to increase their market share and profit margins. Hence, characterization of raw materials, monitoring of food properties during processing, and inspection of final product is crucial. This is achievable by effective and efficient analytical techniques. Additionally, chemical analysis of food samples is not limited to processed food, it is employed to facilitate quality control of fresh commodities by keeping a check on contaminant level, presence of allergen, and adulteration in food samples [85], thus ensuring safety of foods being consumed. Food analysis is also vital for ensuring compliance with food and trade laws for various food commodities. Chemical properties and characteristics of food include pH, titratable acidity, enzymes, immunoassays, contaminants, and their residues.

1.4.1 pH analysis

pH of food samples is the measure of hydrogen ion concentration. The pH in human body ranges between 7.35–7.45, and even slight alterations can cause severe implications, as different organs function at different optimal pH. Pancreatic enzymes function at acidic pH, while enzymes responsible for digestion and absorption of food in intestine require higher or alkaline pH for proper functioning. Thus, pH needs to be maintained. Buffer systems, renal control, and respiratory control are the basic mechanisms responsible for pH control in the human body. Foods establish buffering effect, and the type of food that we intake has a profound impact on the alkalinity/acidity of body fluids. Diet rich in proteins, saturated fats, simple sugars with less fiber, fresh produce, and starchy products, lead to increased acid load, which induces metabolic acidosis [86]. This medical condition clashes with genetically established nutritional needs. Hence, pH analysis of foods being consumed is essential, and consumption of acidic foods, mainly meat and meat products, dairy products, and carbonated drinks should be avoided. The pH of foods affects not only human health but also the food safety. Growth of microorganisms in foods is the major cause of food spoilage, and microbial growth in a specific food depends on its hydronium ion concentration. Increased acidity prevents growth of most microbes, and hence, acidulants are used as food preservatives [87]. Also, pH has an important role to play in food processing. Activity of enzymes is pH-sensitive, and the acidity of sugar solution in jam and jelly preparation needs to be monitored to make high-quality product. Moreover, pH control during juice clarification is mandatory. Thus, constant pH measurement is indispensable to control process variations and produce food products of reliable quality [88].

Mathematically, pH is defined as negative logarithm of hydrogen ion concentration, that is, if the concentration of hydrogen ions is 1×10^{-6}, it is expressed as pH 6. pH scale ranges from 0 to 14, where 0–6, 7, and 8–14 cover acidic, neutral, and basic range, respectively. In modern food analysis, pH is normally assessed instrumentally using a pH meter; however, chemical pH indicators are also available [87]. Chemical indicators largely provide only qualitative information, hence mostly used when pH range of foods needs to be determined. In contrast to this, pH meters provide exact pH readings for all food samples. They work on the principle of potentiometry, wherein an electrolytic cell comprising two electrodes is immersed in a test solution. A voltage proportional to ionic concentration develops, which is measured. This measured voltage is correlated with the pH of solution.

1.4.2 Enzyme analysis

Enzymes are proteinaceous biocatalysts with high specificity and reactivity under optimal physiological conditions. Because most of the enzymes are naturally present in food products, they are thought to be nontoxic and of no concern to consumers. However, food enzymes generated industrially by extraction from plant and animal tissues or fermentation of microorganisms are evaluated for safety. Certain countries like the US and Japan have commercially available digestive enzymes and therapeutic digestive enzymes but are sold as dietary supplements and drugs at the drug store, owing to country-specific regulations and presence of genetically modified enzymes [89]. The effect of industrially generated enzymes on human health is being studied widely. Again, enzymes have wide application in food processing industry, mainly used for juice clarification and peeling of fruits in food industry, improvement of baking quality, and textural quality of flour products, removal of lactose from dairy products, and refinement of quality of meat and meat products [90], making enzyme analysis an integral part of food analysis. Enzymatic analysis refers to the evaluation of chemicals using added enzymes or the measurement of endogenous enzyme activity to provide status of the biological system, and because enzyme catalysis may occur under relatively mild circumstances, it enables for the detection of relatively unstable chemicals that would not be suitable for other methods. Furthermore, the specificity of enzyme reactions allows for the assessment of components of complex mixtures without the time and expense of expensive chromatographic separation procedures [91].

Enzyme activity is a valuable indicator of how well a food product has been processed. The thermal stability of enzymes has been widely utilized as a test of heat treatment; for example, peroxidase activity is used to assess the adequacy of vegetable blanching and phosphatase test to check adequacy of milk pasteurization [92]. Also, food technologists utilize enzyme activity tests to evaluate the efficacy of enzyme preparations used as processing aids. Commercially available enzymes can be used for this purpose. For instance, glucose content in a complex food matrix comprising various monosaccharides can be assessed by using commercially available enzymes. Again, it is employed to assess enzyme activity as a function of enzyme inhibitor content in a diet, as organophosphate insecticides are strong inhibitors of the enzyme acetylcholinesterase; the activity of this enzyme in the presence of a food extract is a good indicator of the organophosphate pesticide concentration in the food [93]. Analysis of enzyme activity also facilitates assessment of food quality, like in the case of catalase, activity is found to increase remarkably in milk from mastitis udders. Additionally, enzymes are also utilized as preparative tools in food analysis. Examples include the employment of amylases and proteases in fiber analysis [94] and the enzymatic hydrolysis of thiamine phosphate esters in vitamin analysis [16]. Thus, information of enzyme activity in advance is vital.

It is required to be familiar with the reaction measuring methods in order to do practical enzyme analysis. Any physical or chemical parameter of the system relating to substrate or product concentration can be employed to track an enzyme reaction. A broad range of techniques for studying enzyme reactions are available, including manometric method, absorbance spectrometry, mass spectrometry, titration, fluorimetry, isotope measurement, chromatography, and viscosity measurements. The spectra of the pyridine coenzymes NAD(H) and NADP(H), in which there is a notable shift in absorbance at 340 nm during oxidation–reduction, are an excellent illustration of the use of spectrophotometry as a tool for tracking enzyme activities. When these coenzymes are products or substrates in a coupled process, several approaches rely on the rise or reduction in absorbance at 340 nm [91].

α-amylase is an endoenzyme that cleaves starch at −1,4 bonds, an example of employing many techniques to quantify the activity of an enzyme. This reaction can be studied by a variety of ways, including viscosity decrease, color reduction of the starch iodine complex increased reducing groups upon hydrolysis, and polarimetry. However, using a single test, it is difficult to distinguish the activity of α-amylase from β-amylase. The former's activity induces a significant drop in starch viscosity and a reduction in iodine color, while the latter may also cause changes in viscosity and iodine color if present in large concentrations [94]. The analyst must evaluate the change in number of reducing groups as a basis of comparison to determine whether β-amylase or α-amylase is being measured as α-amylase is an endoenzyme, which causes bond near center of polymeric substrate to hydrolyze resulting in a significant drop in viscosity, while β-amylase being exoenzyme, hydrolyzes equal number of bonds, without effecting the viscosity of test solution. When creating an enzyme assay, it is best to start with a comprehensive, balanced equation for the specific enzyme-catalyzed reaction. Inspection of the products and substrates for chemical and physical features that are easily measured using widely accessible equipment can frequently result in an evident strategy for following the reaction in the laboratory. If there are several methodologies available, one needs to choose a methodology that can continually monitor the reaction, is specific for the enzyme-catalyzed reaction, and is most sensitive [91].

1.4.3 Food contaminants analysis

The food supply system, which begins with farmers' doorstep and finishes with consumers' plates, is a complex chain, indulges various stages of production and distribution process like planting, harvesting, transporting, storing, importing, processing, packaging, and distribution to retail shops and shelf storing. Various food practices take place at each stage in the food supply chain system, for instance, pesticide treatments to protect crops from pests, weeds or diseases, and humans from vector-borne diseases, such as malaria, dengue fever, etc. Agricultural bioengineering, environmental and storage situations are important factors for product shelf-life, utilization of food additives, selection criteria for food packaging material, and many more. Each of these steps is significant to enhance food safety and quality protocol according to legislation and regulations [95]. Moreover, it is also essential to provide information about rules and regulation to farmers/consumers and the food industry for food contaminants and residues analysis. Here, food quality plays a significant role in analyzing all residues and allows only Food and Drug Administration (FDA)-approved range of food products to be sold in the market. The focused issue is about whether an adverse effect of contaminants is directly related to the dose range; therefore, for each additive found in the product, tolerance value or threshold value must be specified. The EPA (US Environmental Protection Agency) is responsible for creating these tolerance values or ranges and FDA and USDA (United States Department of Agriculture) enforces them publicly.

According to the rapid alert system for food and feed (RASFF), contaminants can be categorized under different compounds such as food allergens (sulfite and histamine), heavy metals (mercury/lead/cadmium), pesticides (omethoate/dimethoate/isofenphos-methyl), veterinary drugs (beta-lactam/nitrofurans/sulfonamide/chloramphenicol), and microbial residues including molds/viruses/bacteria. Some other chemical hazards are used in fraud and food adulterants (melamine), and they are also present in packaging material (bisphenol A/4-methylbenzophenone). Discussed content has strong concerns regarding their impact on human health. Therefore, adequate and feasible methods are used to detect and analyze food contaminants to ensure food quality and safety of individual food products, which travel from agricultural ground to consumer gut. This following section covers the screening methods used for the detection and qualification of food hazards [96].

1.4.3.1 Pesticide analysis

The research findings estimated approximately 800 active molecules belonging to different chemical groups that are used in formulating pesticide product [97]. Pesticides are the compounds responsible for killing pests and broadly classified as herbicides (triazine and atrazine), insecticides (organochlorine, dichloro diphenyl trichloro ethane, organophosphates, and methyl carbamates) and fungicides (phthalimide, captan) [98].

Pesticides not only protect the crop from being wasted but are also essential in protecting humans from various diseases caused by pests. However, they may also have adverse effect on human health, for example, cancer, chronic neurodevelopmental impairment, acute neurologic toxicity, dysfunction of the immune system, etc. [99] Therefore, to monitor their use, tolerance values set up by the FDA are used as a basis all over the world. EPA uses risk assessment studies to determine the toxic effect of pesticide compounds and to establish the range at which no side effects are reported on human health called NOAEL (no observed adverse effect level). The accepted range is known as ADI, that is, acceptable daily intake for humans and can be calculated by using a safety factor of 100 (ADI = NOAEL/100). In Table 1.4, different analytical techniques are applied to detect pesticide analytes with their operating principle. To monitor pesticide, enzyme inhibition assay principle is to inhibit esterase activity in insects that can change the color and be used for detection of organophosphate compounds (malathion, diazinon, and parathion) in fruits, vegetables, and dairy and meat products. If organophosphate is present in food above tolerance level, it may cause headache, fatigue, extremities tingling, and it is also associated with the normal depression in cholinesterase activity [100,101].

Immunoassay method has been used to detect specific compounds using hapten—protein conjugation principle. Haptens are electrophilic in nature and covalently bind to nucleophilic residues on endogenous protein to form a novel antigenic epitope and help in examining the interaction between pesticides analytes. The presence of acylodien insecticide in rice, wheat, and maize using hapten—protein conjugation is essential because if it is present in above tolerance level, it may cause several side effects to human beings, such as dermatological issues, gastrointestinal, neurological, carcinogenic in nature, reproductive as well as endocrine effects [102,103]. Other techniques also play a significant role in pesticide analysis in food products, for example, thin layer chromatography to detect orthophosphates [104,105] and HPLC to analyze urea, benzoylurea, and N-methyl carbamate [106,107] as shown in Table 1.8. Therefore, pesticide analysis has to be applied under strict protocols to avoid above-mentioned health issues and promote food quality and safety standards.

Table 1.8 Analytical techniques used to detect contaminant residues.

Analytical technique	Contaminants residues	Operating principle	Application	Human Health Complaints	Reference
Pesticide analysis					
Enzyme inhibition	Malathion, diazinon, parathion	Inhibition of specific enzyme (if pesticide is present, no change in color)	Water, grains, fruits, vegetables, dairy, and meat products	Headache, dizziness, breathing issues, abdominal cramps, etc.	[100,101]
Immunoassay	Acylodien insecticide, triazine herbicide	Work as class or compound specific interaction (hapten–protein conjugate)	Fruits and vegetables, rice, wheat, maize	Demagogical, gastrointestinal, neurological effects	[102,103]
Thin-layer chromatography	Orthophosphates, carbamate, carbendazim	Semiquantitative method	Kale leaves, orange juice	Embryotoxicity, apoptosis, teratogenicity, infertility	[104,105]
HPLC	NMC, urea, benzoylurea, benzimidazole	Separation based on three parameters samples distribution between mobile and stationary phase	Edible fungi, fruit, fish, vegetables, meat	Low acute toxicity, nausea, vomiting	[106,107]
Mycotoxin analysis					
RIA	Mycotoxin (aflatoxin)	Use of radiolabeled molecules to form immune complex and measure concentration of substances	Meat, soybean, rice, maize	Liver cancer, alteration in protein metabolism, respiratory issues	[97,108]

Lateral flow receptor	Aflatoxin M1/M2, Deoxynivalenol (DON)/OCT/ Zearalenone	Immuno-chromatographic test	Milk, grain, grape juice, feedstuffs, wine	Hepatotoxicity, teratotoxicity, abdominal pain	[109,110]
Immunoaffinity columns with HPLC	Fumonisin, aflatoxin M1/M2	Quantitative method and combination of IAC with HPLC	Milk products, wheat, grains, coffee, nuts	Diarrhea, abdominal pain, esophageal cancer	[109,111]
HPLC	Patulin, sterigmatocystin, zearalenone, DON	Used for quantitative determination	Fruit juices, oats, corn, nuts, wine, coffee	Nausea, lung congestion, carcinogenic, immunosuppressive	[109,112]

1.4.3.2 Mycotoxin analysis

Food products are highly susceptible to mold development under uncontrolled conditions. The growth of fungal species belonging to the genera of *Fusarium, Aspergillus, and Penicillium* produces different types of chemically derived toxins, known as mycotoxins. The attack of mycotoxin on crops can be provoked by environmental factors such as humidity, temperature, mechanical damage of kernels, attack of pests, and fluctuation in weather. In addition, other factors like plant stress caused by extreme soil dryness and unbalanced nutrient absorptions are also responsible for giving space for fungal growth and becoming part of the food supply chain. According to the United Nations Food and Agriculture Organization, up to 25% of the world total crop plants per year are adversely affected by unacceptable levels of mycotoxins [109]. According to the major toxicological classification of mycotoxin, its impact on human health indulges aflatoxins; B1, B2, M1, M2, G1, and G2, and ochratoxin A. The adverse effect of mycotoxin causes genotoxicity, mutagenicity, carcinogenicity, and immunotoxicity. There are some facts regarding tolerance level of mycotoxins present in food products, but unfortunately for aflatoxin B1, no such postulate threshold dose or safe dose range has been created by food organizations. The limit range of mycotoxin exposure to human health is a significant step to avoid the presence of unacceptable mycotoxin level in food products. Therefore, periodic testing protocols become a necessary footstep with proper adoption of sampling procedures and authenticated methods of analysis. Some organizations play a specific role in method validation for mycotoxin analysis: AOCS International, AOCS (American Oil Chemists Society), and AACC International. Table 1.8 provides collective information about techniques availed to examine mycotoxin residues in food. Radioimmunoassay has been reported to be applied to detect mycotoxin (aflatoxin) in maize, soyabean, rice, etc. [108]. Additionally, different techniques including use of lateral flow receptors [110], immunoaffinity columns with HPLC [111], and HPLC [112] are also employed for the analysis of various mycotoxins in food matrices like juice, wine, milk, and nuts.

1.5 Importance of food analysis in relation to COVID-19

The presence of pathogens in the food supply chain has always been a critical issue for managing food safety and quality, epidemic prevention, and public healthcare management. However, the viral epidemics are less discussed and reported as compared to the bacteria, although their transferability rate is very high. With the outbreak of coronavirus disease in 2019 (COVID-19), detection of viral contamination in food samples has become a highly significant. Nevertheless, WHO, EFSA (European Food Safety Authority), and CDC (Centre for Disease Control and Prevention) have claimed that in respect to COVID-19, there is no indication that food poses a risk to public health [113–115]. COVID-19 is mostly transmitted from person to person, primarily by respiratory droplets produced when infected persons sneeze, cough, or blow. As these droplets are rather heavy to hang in the air, they would fall swiftly on floors or surfaces. Infection can occur via breathing in the virus if one is within 1 m of a person infected with COVID-19, or by touching a contaminated surface and then touching one's eyes, nose, or mouth before washing one's hands. In addition, consuming contaminated food may allow the infectious virus to enter the human body (Fig. 1.6). However, processed and packaged foods may pose a risk since the surface of packing material may contain SARS-CoV-2, possibly as a result of contamination by food handlers.

The evidence of SARS-CoV-2 presence on the solid surface (plastic) is reported, and its viability is longer than 72 h. Wet food market has become more prone to providing shelter to SARS-CoV-2 virus as it is positively present in cold chain foods in China. Low temperatures are proven to

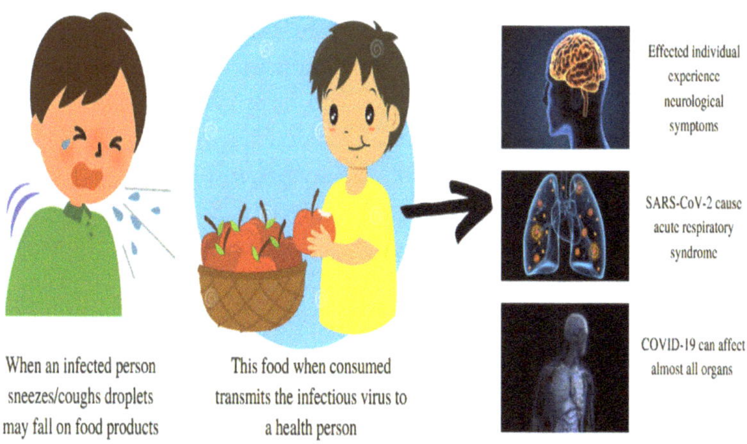

Figure 1.6 Schematic diagram for possible way of SARS-CoV-2 transmission through food.

enhance viral survival, as Fisher et al. in 2020 revealed that SARS-CoV-2 may persist on frozen and refrigerated meat and salmon for more than three weeks [116]. Similar findings were reported by Harbourt et al. The virus was found to be stable on swine skin for 14 days, 96 h, and 8 h at 4°C, 22°C, and 37°C, respectively [117]. Taking this into account, the authors theorized that the virus may be transferred across locations and infect employees and handlers through cold chain supply and storage of foods. Although low-temperature storage is favorable for viral contamination, cooking drastically reduces the infection levels in food. ANSES, the French agency for food, environmental, and occupational health and safety claimed that cooking food for only 4 min at 63°C might reduce the SARS-CoV-2 contamination level in food product by 1000 times [118]. Thus, contaminated food and food packaging material are not that potent transmitters of the virus if they are handled carefully and by following the guidelines issued by various health organizations across the globe.

1.5.1 Food safety management in COVID-19 era

With the outbreak of COVID-19, the food system has been exposed to an unknown danger. However, it is critical that customers maintain their faith in food safety. The FDA and the WHO proposed additional steps to ensure food safety and the integrity of the food chain in the COVID-19 period. Primarily, the critical importance of limited close contact in food manufacturing facilities has been highlighted [119]. Human contact with food bears major risk of contamination of food commodities. Hence, it was recommended that food handlers should keep their masks and gloves on while handling food and change them frequently. Also, hand sanitization was included in hand hygiene guidelines to limit the infectivity and spread of the pathogenic virus. WHO recommended use of hand sanitizers with the formulations of ethanol, glycerol, and hydrogen peroxide (80, 1.45, and 0.125% v/v, respectively) or 2-propanol, glycerol, and hydrogen peroxide (75, 1.45 and 0.125% v/v, respectively). These hand-rub sanitizers are reported to effectively inactivate SARS-CoV-2 in 30 s [120]. Ensuring food safety is not the only goal; the most difficult task for food industry is to safeguard food workers from getting infected with COVID-19, to avoid viral exposure or transmission, and to improve food hygiene and sanitation measures. For this, maintaining physical distancing among food handlers is critical. Thus, the reduction in number of workers in food industry was suggested relying more on frequently sanitized automated machines.

Also, noncontact delivery of food and essential items were recommended. With this, the cleaning and sanitization of all bags used for food delivery became essential. As food delivery is not always feasible, it was recommended that the retail stores should maintain a safe atmosphere to safeguard workers and customers from getting infected [121]. Controlling the number of clients who enter the retail business is good for avoiding overcrowding and facilitating physical separation. Wipes, hand sanitizers, and disinfectant sprays are available at shop entrance points to reduce the risk of contact and illness. And to manage open food hygienically, WHO recommended plexiglass installation to avoid touch or placing it in plastic/cellophane or paper packaging. All surfaces in touch with food should be cleaned on a regular basis, and everyone in the open food area (customers or employees) should maintain proper personal hygiene. It is critical that the food that consumers consume is safe, and hence, WHO advised washing of fruits and vegetables thoroughly with portable water before consumption. Also, foods must be adequately cooked, as thermal processing strongly reduce the infectivity of the virus, if at all it is present [122]. In addition to the above recommendations, several other guidelines have been issued to aid the food business, ensure food safety, and consumer health during this critical COVID-19 era. The most relevant guidelines issued by competent authorities are summarized in the Table 1.9.

1.5.2 SARS-CoV-2 virus analysis

Although it is claimed that food is not health hazard in relation to COVID-19, it is still essential to detect its presence in cold chain supply system. In cold storage places and transportation, temperature is below 0°C, which favors adequate growth and longer survival time of the virus on packaging material. Therefore, fast and sensitive methods with feasibility cost are essential for detection COVID-19 in cold-chain foods. SARS-CoV-2 virions have tendency to bind with its receptor having spike protein on its surface and S1 subunit works as the receptor-binding domain. Therefore, S1 subunit was selected as the biomarker for SARS-CoV-2 detection and analytical technique used to detect its interdigitated microelectrode chip (IDME). In this anti-SARS-CoV-2 S-protein Ab (antibody) is immobilized on an IDME chip and then AC (alternating signal) is sent to induce an electrophoresis force on the protein substance. Therefore, S-protein comes toward the IDME surface in the nanofluid and is attached to the antibodies [138]. Thermo Fisher Scientific is

Table 1.9 Summary of food industry related guidelines in COVID-19 era.

Guidelines	Issuing authority	References
Guidelines for food safety		
COVID-19 and food Safety: Guidance for food businesses interim guidanceCOVID-19: Animal–human interface and food safety	WHO	[113]
COVID-19 and food safety: Guidance for competent authorities responsible for national food safety control systems interim guidanceCOVID-19: Animal–human interface and food safety	WHO	[122]
WHO recommendations to reduce risk of transmission of emerging pathogens from animals to humans in live animal markets or animal product marketsCOVID-19: Animal–human interface and food safety	WHO	[123]
COVID-19 information for consumers shopping for food	FDA	[124]
Temporary policy during the COVID-19 public health emergency regarding the qualified exemption from the standards for the growing, harvesting, packing, and holding of produce for human consumption	FDA	[125]
Best practices for retail food stores, restaurants, and food pick-up/delivery services during the COVID-19 pandemic	FDA	[126]
Guidelines for Hygiene Practices		
Recommendations to member states to improve hand hygiene practices to help prevent the transmission of the COVID-19 virus	WHO	[127]
Guide to local production: WHO recommended hand rub formulations	WHO	[128]
Advice on the use of masks in the context of COVID-19	WHO	[129]
Proper usage of face masks/coverings to protect against COVID-19	FDA	[130]
Guidelines for GMPs and GHPs in food industries		
Water, sanitation, hygiene, and waste management for SARS-CoV-2, the virus that causes COVID-19	WHO	[131]

(*Continued*)

Table 1.9 (Continued)

Guidelines	**Issuing authority**	**References**
Food and agriculture: Considerations for Prioritization of PPE, cloth Face coverings, disinfectants, and sanitation supplies during the COVID-19 pandemic	FDA	[132]
Cleaning and disinfection of environmental surfaces in the context of COVID-19	WHO	[133]
Best practices for reopening retail food establishments during the COVID-19 pandemic-food safety checklist	FDA	[134]
Employee health and food safety checklist for human and animal food operations during the COVID-19 pandemic	FDA; OSHA	[135]
Protecting seafood processing workers from COVID-19 seafood processing workers	CDC; FDA; OSHA	[136]
meat and poultry processing workers and employers	CDC; OSHA	[137]

HPLC: High-performance liquid chromatography; *NMC*: N-methyl carbamate; *RIA*: radioimmunoassay; *FPIA*: Fluorescence polarization immunoassay; *DON*; Deoxynivalenol; *GHP*; Good Hygienic Practice.

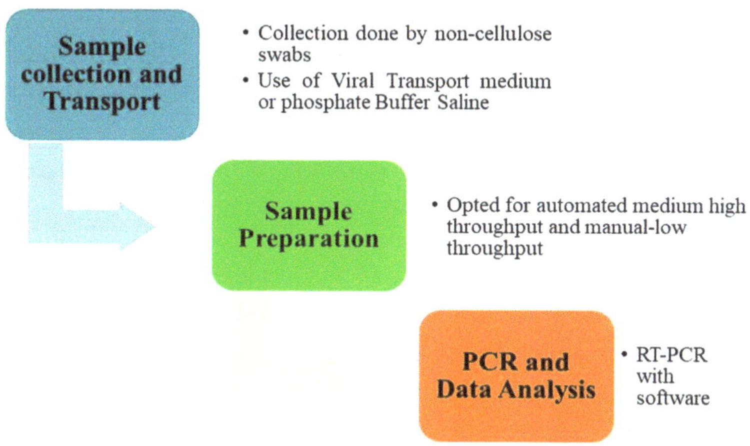

Figure 1.7 Workflow of detection of SARS-CoV-2 on food packaging.

continuously working on developing analytical techniques to detect SARS-CoV-2 in an effective way. Studies have shown that virus can remain viable on common surface like food packaging, for up to 28 days as shown in Fig. 1.7 [139], and virus can be transmitted when a healthy person comes in contact with contaminated space (food or environment including packaging material), and after that touches their mouth, eyes, or nose. Therefore, Thermo Fisher Scientific promotes use of the Quant Studio 5 and 7500 Food safety Fast RT-PCR (real-time polymerase chain reaction) in the detection of SARS-CoV-2 in food samples, packaging, and environment.

1.6 Future prospects

Food analysis is constantly seeking the development of more robust, efficient, sensitive, and cost-effective analytical techniques to ensure food safety, quality, and traceability in accordance with regulations and customer needs. Significant breakthroughs have been made in the last decade. One of the most active areas of study in analytical chemistry, particularly in the food sector, has been the development of new ways of sample preparation and separation techniques. This includes the development and use of molecularly imprinted polymers in food sample analysis, the use of monoliths in milk sample preparation, the use of hydrophilic interaction liquid chromatography (HILIC), and electro-driven separation techniques such as capillary electrophoresis (CE) or microchip capillary electrophoresis and so on. However, these techniques require specialized machinery, which are quite expensive, and therefore, practical research is required in this field to develop portable and economic machinery. Moreover, the use of biological techniques is still at growing stage, although DNA-based techniques, biosensors, and molecular methods are the few advances that lead to major developments in this field. Hence, advanced study is required in this promising sector. Also, toxic residues in food are becoming more prevalent as a result of industrial expansion, new farming techniques, environmental degradation, and climate change. This causes significant difficulty in detection of untargeted substances and determination of their identification in foods, and thus, there is a need for developing new analytical tools. Despite these significant advances, hundreds of food-borne infection cases continue to occur across the world, and up to one-third of the population in developed countries suffers from food-borne sickness each year. Microbiologists have developed viable culture-based approaches for pathogen detection in foods during the last few decades. These approaches are considered the "gold standard," although they are time-consuming and inconvenient and hence require enhancements. There is also a lot of discussion on how to assure global food safety and the multiple roles of risk analysis, including microbiological risk assessment. In this sense, benefit–risk evaluation in food and nutrition considers both the positive and negative effects that a food (component) may have in order to support better informed management decisions addressing public health concerns. The use of nanoparticles in food science is suitable to explore through benefit–risk analysis. Nanotechnology and nanomaterials have the potential to significantly improve food supply through novel applications such as nutrient and bioactive absorption and delivery systems, microbial, allergen, and contaminant detection and control, food packaging properties and performance, and improved colors and flavors. Also, additional toxicological research on various types of nanomaterials is required to understand how they might affect food safety, and more appropriate analytical approaches for detecting allergens in foods are still necessary, because even trace levels of the allergen can have serious implications in sensitive people. Besides, major advances in food supply chain management are required. The farmers should have the provision to monitor the quality of raw material to facilitate production of high-quality food product ultimately. Therefore, portable analytical equipment required to assess the food quality and safety parameters should be designed. Furthermore, to reduce the amount of toxic chemicals produced during analysis, the inception of concept of green chemistry came into being; however, the implementation of green analytical chemistry in food analysis laboratories is a significant challenge, and as a result, suitable approaches are constantly being considered.

1.7 Conclusions

Food composition and characteristics must be investigated in order to achieve standard quality products, ensure compliance to food authority recommendations, and provide accurate nutritional labeling in processed food products. Not only is food analysis important, but so is the characterization of various food samples and the selection of sampling techniques. Also, analysis of food includes both chemical and compositional analysis.

Food components such as moisture, fat, protein, carbohydrate, vitamins, and minerals are studied because of their functional importance and impact on food safety and human health. Food chemical analysis includes pH analysis, enzyme kinetics research, and the effect of mycotoxins and pesticide residues in food. A variety of analytical techniques for food samples are also listed including both traditional and modern methods such as HPLC, spectroscopic techniques, radiometric techniques, and chromatographic techniques. Furthermore, with the advent of the COVID-19, the importance of food safety and the impact of undesirable food constituents on human health have multiplied many folds, necessitating the critical need for COVID analysis, as SARS-CoV-2 virus may infiltrate the food chain during food storage and transportation. Hence, detection of viral contamination in food samples is also important for human health in the coming era.

References

[1] Statista Inc. New York United states. *Food consumer market worldwide*, Available from: https://www.statista.com/outlook/cmo/food/worldwide/; 2022 (accessed 31.03.22).
[2] B. Quimby, Detection of toxic industrial compounds: a guide to analytical techniques, Environ. Analysis. AET (2003).
[3] C.M. Galanakis, Functionality of food components and emerging technologies, Foods. 10 (1) (2021) 128.
[4] J.R. Lupien, Prevention and control of food safety risks: the role of governments, food producers, marketers, and academia, Asia Pac. J. Clin. Nutr. 16 (S1) (2007) 74–79.
[5] D.M. Barrett, J.C. Beaulieu, R. Shewfelt, Color, flavor, texture, and nutritional quality of fresh-cut fruits and vegetables: desirable levels, instrumental and sensory measurement, and the effects of processing, Crit. Rev. Food Sci. Nutr. 50 (5) (2010) 369–389.
[6] B. Flickinger, Challenges and solutions in compositional analysis, Food Qual. 3 (19) (1997) 21–26.
[7] S.S. Nielsen, Introduction to food analysis, Food Analysis, Springer, Cham, 2017, pp. 3–16.
[8] P.A. Curtis, Guide to Food Laws and Regulations, Blackwell, 2005.
[9] E.T. Guarino, J. Kellam, International Food Law, Prospect Media, St Leonards, NSW, 2000.
[10] C.N. Murphy, J. Yates, The International Organization for Standardization (ISO): Global Governance through Voluntary Consensus, Routledge, 2009.
[11] Joint FAO/WHO Expert Committee on Food Additives, Combined Compendium of Food Additive Specifications: Analytical Methods, Test Procedures and Laboratory Solutions Used by and Referenced in Food Additive Specifications, Food & Agriculture Org, 2005.
[12] Y. Pomeranz (Ed.), Food Analysis: Theory and Practice, Springer Science & Business Media, 2013.
[13] S. Otles, Handbook of Food Analysis Instruments, CRC Press, 2016.

[14] I. Elmadfa, A.L. Meyer, Importance of food composition data to nutrition and public health, Eur. J. Clin. Nutr. 64 (3) (2010) S4–S7.
[15] L.W. Aurand, A.E. Woods, M.R. Wells, The vitamins, Food Composition and Analysis, Springer, Dordrecht, 1987, pp. 349–417.
[16] AOAC International Official methods of analysis, AOAC International, Gaithersburg, MD 18th edn. Current through revision 2, 2007 (On-line).
[17] H.M. Wehr, J.F. Frank, American Public Health Association, Standard Methods for the Examination of Dairy Products, American Public Health Association;, Washington, DC, 2004.
[18] J. Mitchell Jr, D.M. Smith, Aquametry, Wiley, New York, 1948.
[19] R.L. Bradley, Moisture and total solids analysis, Food Analysis, Springer, Boston, MA, 2010, pp. 85–104.
[20] J. Giese, In-line sensors for food processing, Food Technol. 47 (5) (1993) 87–95.
[21] R.H. Wilson, E.K. Kemsley, On-line process monitoring using infrared techniques, Food Processing Automation II. Proceedings of the American society of agricultural engineers, ASAE Publication, 1992. 02–92. American Society of Agricultural Engineers, St. Joseph, MI.
[22] M. Bockisch, The importance of fats, Fats and Oils Handbook, Elsevier, 1998, pp. 1–52. Available from: http://doi.org/10.1016/b978-0-9818936-0-0.50006-8.
[23] A. Ascherio, W.C. Willett, Health effects of trans fatty acids, Am. J. Clin. Nutr. 66 (4) (1997) 1006–1010.
[24] A.G. Liu, N.A. Ford, F.B. Hu, et al., A healthy approach to dietary fats: understanding the science and taking action to reduce consumer confusion, Nutr. J. 16 (2017) 53.
[25] R.J. Marshall, Combined instrumental and sensory measurement of the role of fat in food texture, Food Qual. Prefer. 2 (2) (1990) 117–124.
[26] S. Bayarri, A.J. Taylor, J. Hort, The role of fat in flavor perception: effect of partition and viscosity in model emulsions, J. Agric. Food Chem. 54 (23) (2006) 8862–8868.
[27] D.B. Min, W.C. Ellefson, Fat analysis, Food Analysis, Springer, Boston, MA, 2010, pp. 117–132.
[28] Joslyn, M. Methods in Food Analysis, second ed. Academic, New York 7.
[29] Y. Pomeranz, C.F. Meloan, Food Analysis: Theory and Practice, third ed., Van Nostrand Reinhold, New York, 1994.
[30] H.M. Wehr, J.F. Frank (Eds.), Standard Methods for the Examination of Dairy Products, seventeenth ed., American Public Health Association, Washington, DC, 2004.
[31] D.A. Cronin, K. McKenzie, A rapid method for the determination of fat in foodstuffs by infrared spectrometry, Food Chem. 35 (1990) 39–49.
[32] J.D. Pettinati, C.E. Swift, Rapid determination of fat in meat and meat products by foss-let solvent extraction and density measurement, J. Assoc. Off. Anal. Chem. 58 (6) (1975) 1182–1187.
[33] S.T.H. Sherazi, S.A. Mahesar, Analysis of edible oils and fats by nuclear magnetic resonance (NMR) spectroscopy, Applications of NMR Spectroscopy, Bentham Science Publishers, 2015, pp. 57–92.
[34] S. Damodaran, Amino acids, peptides and proteins, Fennema's Food Chemistry, 4, CRC Press, 2008, pp. 217–330.
[35] I. Delimaris, Adverse effects associated with protein intake above the recommended dietary allowance for adults, ISRN Nutr. 2013 (2013) 126929.
[36] P.J. Fellows, Properties of food and principles of processing, Food Processing Technology, Woodhead Publishing, 2017, pp. 3–400.
[37] S.K. Chang, Y. Zhang, Protein analysis, Food Analysis, Springer, Cham, 2017, pp. 315–331.

[38] R.B. Bradstreet, The Kjeldahl Method for Organic Nitrogen, Academic, New York, 1965.

[39] P.R. Wilson, A new instument concept for nitrogen/protein analysis. A challenge to the Kjeldahl method, Asp. Appl. Biol. 25 (1990) 443–446.

[40] H.J. Luinge, E. Hop, E.T.G. Lutz, J.A. van Hemert, E.A.M. de Jong, Determination of the fat, protein and lactose content of milk using Fourier transform infrared spectrometry, Anal. Chim. Acta 284 (1993) 419–433.

[41] P.G. Krishnan, W.J. Park, K.D. Kephart, D.L. Reeves, G.L. Yarrow, Measurement of protein and oil content of oat cultivars using near-infrared reflectance, Cereal Foods World 39 (2) (1993) 105–108.

[42] O.H. Lowry, N.J. Rosebrough, A.L. Farr, R.J. Randall, Protein measurement with the Folin phenol reagent, J. Biol. Chem 193 (1951) 265–275.

[43] P.K. Smith, R.L. Krohn, G.T. Hermanson, A.K. Mallia, F.H. Gartner, M.D. Provensano, et al., Measurement of proteinusing bicinchoninic acid, Anal. Biochem 150 (1985) 76–85.

[44] H. Fraenkel-Conrat, M. Cooper, The use of dye for the determination of acid and basic groups in proteins, J. Biol. Chem 154 (1944) 239–246.

[45] M. Bradford, A rapid and sensitive method for the quantitation of microgram quantities of protein utilizing the principle of protein–dye binding, Anal. Biochem 72 (1976) 248–254.

[46] S. Nakai, H.K. Wilson, E.O. Herreid, Spectrophotometric determination of protein in milk, J. Dairy. Sci. (1965) 356–358.

[47] E. Gabor, Determination of the protein content of certain meat products by ultraviolet absorption spectrophotometry, Acta Alimentaria 8 (2) (1979) 157–167.

[48] H.W. Robinson, C.G. Hodgen, The biuret reaction in the determination of serum protein. 1. A study of the conditions necessary for the production of the stable color which bears a quantitative relationship to the protein concentration, J. Biol. Chem. 135 (1950) 707–725.

[49] A.J. Pinckney, The biuret test as applied to the estimation of wheat protein, Cereal Chem. 38 (1961) 501–506.

[50] N. James, BeMiller, K.C. Huber, Carbohydrates, Fennema's Food Chemistry, 4, CRC Press, 2008, pp. 83–155.

[51] X.L. Dong, F. Guan, S.J. Xu, L.X. Zhu, P.P. Zhang, A.B. Cheng, et al., Influence of blood glucose level on the prognosis of patients with diabetes mellitus complicated with ischemic stroke, J. Res. Med. Sci. 23 (2018) 10.

[52] J.N. BeMiller, Carbohydrate analysis, Food Analysis, Springer, Boston, MA, 2010, pp. 147–177.

[53] A. Klockow, A. Paulus, V. Figueiredo, R. Amado, H.M. Widmer, Determination of carbohydrates in fruit juices by capillary electrophoresis and high-performance liquid chromatography, J. Chromatogr. A 680 (1994) 187.

[54] R.F. Jackson, W.D. Chase, J.A. Mathews. *A Analytical Methods for the Determination of Levulose in Crude Products*. 1932. Available from: https://nvlpubs.nist.gov/nistpubs/jres/9/jresv9n5p597_A2b.pdf.

[55] S. Ekelund, Determining reducing sugar. A critical study of Munson and Walker general-method, Acta Agric. Suec. 1 (1946) 239–319.

[56] T.G. Ludwig, H.J. Goldberg, The anthrone method for the determination of carbohydrates in foods and in oral rinsing, J. Dental Res. 35 (1) (1956) 90–94.

[57] L.S. Magwaza, U.L. Opara, Analytical methods for determination of sugars and sweetness of horticultural products—a review, Sci. Hortic. 184 (2015) 179–192.

[58] M. Mehrübeoglu, G.L. Coté, Determination of total reducing sugars in potato samples using near-infrared spectroscopy, Cereal Foods World 42 (1997) 409. and references therein.

[59] H. Di Paola, R.D. Asis, R. Aldao, MA. Evaluation of the degree of starch gelatinization by a new enzymatic method, Starch-Stärke 55 (9) (2003) 403–409.
[60] R.R. Ruan, C. Zou, C. Wadhawan, B. Martinez, P.L. Chen, P. Addis, Studies of hardness and water mobility of cooked wild rice using nuclear magnetic resonance 1, J. Food Process. Preservation 21 (2) (1997) 91–104.
[61] B. Conde-Petit, F. Escher, Influence of starch-lipid complexation on the ageing behaviour of high concentration starch gels, Starch-Staerke 46 (1994) 172–177.
[62] J. Silverio, E. Svensson, A.C. Eliasson, G. Olofsson, Isothermal microcalorimetric studies on starch retrogradation, J. Therm. Anal. Calorim. 47 (5) (1996) 1179–1200.
[63] C.H. Teo, C.C. Seow, A pulsed NMR method for the study of starch retrogradation, Starch-Stärke 44 (8) (1992) 288–292.
[64] K.R. Morgan, R.H. Furneaux, R.A. Stanley, Observation by solid-state 3C CP MAS NMR spectroscopy of the transformations of wheat starch associated with the making and staling of bread, Carbohydr. Res. 235 (1992) 15–22.
[65] N. Thiex, Evaluation of analytical methods for the determination of moisture, crude protein, crude fat, and crude fiber in distillers dried grains with solubles, J. AOAC Int. 92 (1) (2009) 61–73.
[66] F. Jesse, Gregory III, Vitamins, Fennema's Food Chemistry, CRC Press, 2008, pp. 439–522.
[67] R.B. Pegg, W.O. Landen, R.R. Eitenmiller, Vitamin analysis, Food Analysis, Springer, Boston, MA, 2010, pp. 179–200.
[68] G.L. Newton, R.E. Tucker, G.E. Mitchell Jr, G.T. Schelling, N.E. Alderson, W.M. Knight, Bioassay of vitamin A in liquid supplements, J. Int. de. Vitaminologie et. de Nutrition. 49 (3) (1979) 240–245.
[69] T.C. Stamp, J.G. Haddad Jr, A.N. Exton-Smith, A. Reuben, C.A. Twigg, Assay of vitamin D and its metabolites, Ann. Clin. Biochem. 13 (1-6) (1976) 571–577.
[70] J.G. Bell, Microbiological assay of vitamins of the B group in foodstuffs, Laboratory Pract. 23 (5) (1974) 235–252.
[71] A. Rizzolo, S. Polesello, Chromatographic determination of vitamins in foods, J. Chromatogr. 624 (1-2) (1992) 103–152.
[72] Y. Zhang, W.E. Zhou, J.Q. Yan, M. Liu, Y. Zhou, X. Shen, et al., A Review of the extraction and determination methods of thirteen essential vitamins to the human body: an update from 2010, Molecules (Basel, Switz.) 23 (6) (2018) 1484.
[73] M.F. Md Noh, R.D. Gunasegavan, K.N. Mustafa, V. Balasubramaniam, S. Mustar, Abd, et al., Recent techniques in nutrient analysis for food composition database, Molecules 25 (19) (2020) 4567.
[74] R.B. Roy, A. Conetta, J. Salpeter, Automated fluorometric method for determination of total vitamin C in food products, J. Assoc. Off. Anal. Chem. 59 (6) (1976) 1244–1250.
[75] L. Casella, M. Gullotti, A. Marchesini, M. Petrarulo, Rapid enzymatic method for Vitamin C assay in fruits and vegetables using peroxidase, J. Food Sci. 54 (1989) 374–375.
[76] T.R. Guilarte, B. Shane, P.A. Mcintyre, Radiometric-microbiologic assay of Vitamin B-6: application to food analysis, J. Nutr. 111 (11) (1981) 1869–1875.
[77] D.D. Miller, Minerals, Fennema's Food Chemistry, 4, CRC Press, 2008, pp. 523–570.
[78] R.E. Ward, C.E. Carpenter, Traditional methods for mineral analysis, Food Analysis, Springer, Boston, MA, 2010, pp. 201–215.
[79] A.D. Eaton, L.S. Clesceri, E.W. Rice, A.E. Greenburg, editors. *Standard Methods for the Examination of Water and Wastewater*, 21st edn. Method 2340, hardness. American Public Health Association, American Water Works Association, Water Environment Federation, Washington, DC, 2005, p. 2–37.

[80] Z. Stanić, T. Dimić, Natural mineral pyrite and analytical application thereof in precipitation titrations in non-aqueous solvents, N. J. Chem. 37 (11) (2014) 3612–3619.
[81] C. Carpenter, E. Clark, Evaluation of iron methods used in meat iron analysis and iron content of raw and cooked meats, J. Agric. Food Chem. 43 (1995) 1824–1827.
[82] A.K. Covington (Ed.), Ion Selective Electrode Methodology, CRC, Boca Raton, FL, 1980.
[83] Das S. Chanda, S. Paul, B. Singh, P. Giri, Shiba, Mineral assay in atomic absorption spectroscopy, Beats Nat. Sci. 1 (2014) 1–17.
[84] M.B. Jacobs, The chemical analysis of foods and food products, The Chemical Analysis of Foods and Food Products, third ed., 1951.
[85] R. Anna, A. Zeineb, F. Salvatore, Chiral separations in food analysis, TrAC. Trends Anal. Chem. 52 (2013) 206–225.
[86] G.K. Schwalfenberg, The alkaline diet: is there evidence that an alkaline pH diet benefits health? J. Environ. Public. Health (2012) 727630.
[87] G.D. Sadler, P.A. Murphy, pH and titratable acidity, Food Analysis, Springer, Boston, MA, 2010, pp. 219–238.
[88] P. Vijayakumar, A.A. Adedeji, *Measuring the pH of Food Products*. University of Kentucky. 2017.
[89] Y. Hirose, Enzymes for human nutrition and health, Industrial Enzyme Applications, Wiley, 2019.
[90] P. Fernandes, Enzymes in food processing: a condensed overview on strategies for better biocatalysts, Enzyme Res. 2010 (2010) 862537.
[91] J.R. Powers, Application of enzymes in food analysis, Food Analysis, Springer, Boston, MA, 2010, pp. 283–299.
[92] S.A. Rankin, A. Christiansen, W. Lee, D.S. Banavara, A. Lopez-Hernandez, Invited review: the application of alkaline phosphatase assays for the validation of milk product pasteurization, J. Dairy. Sci. 3 (12) (2010) 5538–5551.
[93] J. Patočka, K. Kuča, D. Jun, Acetylcholinesterase and butyrylcholinesterase–important enzymes of human body, Acta Medica (Hradec Kralove) 47 (4) (2004) 215–228.
[94] P. Bernfeld, Amylases, α and β, Methods Enzymol. 1 (1955) 149–158. AOAC 1:14.
[95] I.S. Arvanitoyannis, International regulations on food contaminants and residues, Compr. Anal. Chem. 51 (2008) 29–76.
[96] M.W. Nielen, H.J. Marvin, Challenges in chemical food contaminants and residue analysis, Compr. Anal. Chem. 51 (2008) 1–27.
[97] G. Miklós, C. Angeli, Á. Ambrus, A. Nagy, V. Kardos, A. Zentai, et al., Detection of aflatoxins in different matrices and food-chain positions, Front. Microbiol 11 (2020) 1916.
[98] B. Ismail, B.L. Reuhs, S.S. Nielsen, Analysis of food contaminants, residues, and chemical constituents of concern, Food Analysis, Springer, Boston, MA, 2010, pp. 317–349.
[99] Y. Picó (Ed.), Wilson & Wilson's Comprehensive Analytical Chemistry: Food Contaminants and Residue Analysis, Elsevier, 2008.
[100] E.D. Richter, P. Chuwers, Y. Levy, M. Gordon, F. Grauer, J. Marzouk, et al., Health effects from exposure to organophosphate pesticides in workers and residents in Israel, Isr. J. Med. Sci. 28 (8-9) (1992) 584–598.
[101] J.L. Tadeo, Analysis of pesticides in food and environmental samples. CRC.
[102] Z. Liu, K. Wang, S. Wu, Z. Wang, G. Ding, X. Hao, et al., Development of an immunoassay for the detection of carbaryl in cereals based on a camelid variable heavy-chain antibody domain, J. Sci. Food Agric. 99 (9) (2019) 4383–4390.

[103] N.A. Lee, I.R. Kennedy, Environmental monitoring of pesticides by immunoanalytical techniques: validation, current status, and future perspectives, J. AOAC Int. 84 (5) (2001) 1393–1406.

[104] Z. Shen, Q. Fan, Q. Yu, R. Wang, H. Wang, X. Kong, Facile detection of carbendazim in food using TLC-SERS on diatomite thin layer chromatography, Spectrochim. Acta A Mol. Biomol. Spectrosc. 247 (2021) 119037.

[105] S. Singh, N. Singh, V. Kumar, S. Datta, A.B. Wani, D. Singh, et al., Toxicity, monitoring and biodegradation of the fungicide carbendazim, Environ. Chem. Lett. 14 (3) (2016) 317–329.

[106] Q. Zeng, J. Zhang, D. Xu, Z. Zhang, Z. Ke, Determination of urea in canned foods by high performance liquid chromatography-fluorescence detection coupled with precolumn derivatization, Se pu = Chin. J. Chromatogr. 33 (1) (2015) 80–83.

[107] B.E. Watt, A.T. Proudfoot, S.M. Bradberry, J.A. Vale, Poisoning due to urea herbicides, Toxicological Rev. 24 (3) (2005) 161–166.

[108] G.S. Shephard, Impact of mycotoxins on human health in developing countries, Food Addit. Contam. 25 (2) (2008) 146–151.

[109] C. Brera, B. De Santis, F. Debegnach, M. Miraglia, MycotoxinsD. Barcelo (ed) in: Y. Pico (Ed.), Food Contaminants and Residue Analysis. Comprehensive Analytical Chemistry, 51, Elsevier, Oxford, UK, 2008.

[110] A. Dhakal, E. Sbar, Aflatoxin Toxicity, StatPearls, 2020.

[111] K.A. Voss, R.T. Riley, N.M. Gardner, J. Gelineau-van Waes, Fumonisins, Reproductive and Developmental Toxicology, Academic Press, 2017, pp. 925–943.

[112] B. Caballero, L.C. Trugo, P.M. Finglas, Encyclopedia of Food Sciences and Nutrition, Academic, 2003.

[113] WHO. *COVID-19 and food safety: Guidance for food businesses: Interim guidance.* Available from: https://www.who.int/publications/i/item/covid-19-and-food-safety-%20guidance-for-food-businesses; 2020 (accessed 19.04.22).

[114] EFSA. *Coronavirus: No evidence that food is a source or transmission route*, 2020. Available from: https://www.efsa.europa.eu/en/news/coronavirus-no-evidence-food-source-or-transmission-route (accessed 19.04.22).

[115] CDC. *Food safety and cornonavirus disease 2019 (COVID-19).* 2020. Available from: https://www.cdc.gov/foodsafety/newsletter/food-safety-and-Coronavirus.html (accessed 19.04.22).

[116] D. Fisher, A. Reilly, A. Kang, E. Zheng, A.R. Cook, D.E. Anderson, Seeding of outbreaks of COVID-19 by contaminated fresh and frozen food, bioRxiv (2020).

[117] D.E. Harbourt, A.D. Haddow, A.E. Piper, H. Bloomfield, B.J. Kearney, D. Fetterer, et al., Modeling the stability of severe acute respiratory syndrome coronavirus 2 (SARS-CoV-1 2) on skin, currency, and clothing, PLoSNegl Trop. Dis. 14 (11) (2020) e0008831.

[118] ANSES. *ANSES's recommendations on food, shopping and cleaning.* Available from: https://www.anses.fr; 2020 (accessed 19.04.22).

[119] X. Pang, L. Ren, S. Wu, W. Ma, J. Yang, L. Di, et al., Cold-chain food contamination as the possible origin of Covid-19 resurgence in Beijing, Natl. Sci. Rev. 7 (2020) 1861–1864.

[120] A. Kratzel, S. Steiner, D. Todt, P. V'kovski, Y. Brueggemann, J. Steinmann, et al., Temperature dependent surface stability of SARS-CoV-2, J. Infect. 81 (2020) 452–482.

[121] G. Kampf, A. Voss, S. Scheithauer, Inactivation of coronaviruses by heat, J. Hosp. Infect. 105 (2020) 348–349.

[122] WHO. *COVID-19 and Food Safety: Guidance for Competent Authorities Responsible for National Food Safety Control Systems.* Available from: https://www.who.int/publications/i/item/covid-19-and-food-safety-guidance-for-competent-authoritiesresponsible-for-national-food-safety-control-systems; 2020 (accessed 19.04.22).

[123] WHO. *Recommendations to Reduce Risk of Transmission of Emerging Pathogens from Animals to Humans in Live Animal Markets*. Available from: https://www.who.int/health-topics/coronavirus/whorecommendations-to-reduce-risk-of-transmission-of-emerging-pathogens-from-animals-to-humans-in-live-animal-markets; 2020 (accessed 19.04.22).
[124] FDA. *Shopping for Food During the COVID-19 Pandemic—Information for Consumers*. Available from: https://www.fda.gov/food/food-safety-during-emergencies/shopping-food-during-covid-19-pandemic-information-consumers; 2020 (accessed 19.04.22).
[125] FDA. *Temporary Policy During the COVID-19 Public Health Emergency Regarding the Qualified Exemption from the Standards for the Growing, Harvesting, Packing, and Holding of Produce for Human Consumption Guidance for Industry*. Available from: https://www.fda.gov/regulatory-information/search-fda-guidance-documents/temporary-policy-during-covid-19-public-health-emergency-regarding-qualified-exemption-standards; 2020 (accessed 19.04.22).
[126] FDA. *Best Practices for Retail Food Stores, Restaurants, and Food Pick-Up/Delivery Services during the COVID-19*. Available form: https://www.fda.gov/food/food-safety-during-emergencies/best-practices-retail-food-stores-restaurants-and-foodpick-updelivery-services-during-covid-19#employeehealth; 2020 (accessed 19.04.22).
[127] WHO. *Recommendations to Member States to Improve Hand Hygiene Practices to Help Prevent the Transmission of the COVID19 Virus*. Available from: https://www.who.int/publications/i/item/recommendations-to-member-states-to-improve-handhygiene-practices-to-help-prevent-the-transmission-of-the-covid-19-virus; 2020 (accessed 19.04.22).
[128] World Health Organization (WHO). *Guide to Local Production: WHO-Recommended Hand rub Formulations Introduction*. Available from: https://www.who.int/gpsc/5may/Guide_to_Local_Production.pdf; 2020 (accessed 19.04.22).
[129] WHO. *Advice on the Use of Masks in the Context of COVID-19: Interim Guidance-2*. Available from: https://apps.who.int/iris/handle/10665/331693; 2020 (accessed 19.04.22).
[130] CDC. *Proper Usage of Face Masks/Coverings to Protect against COVID-19*. Available from: https://www.cdc.gov/coronavirus/%202019-ncov/prevent-getting-sick/cloth-face-cover.html; 2020 (accessed 19.04.22).
[131] WHO. *Water, Sanitation, Hygiene, and Waste Management for SARS-CoV-2, the Virus that Causes COVID-19*. Available from: https://www.who.int/publications/i/item/water-sanitation-hygiene-and-waste-management-for-the-covid-19-virusinterim-guidance; 2020 (accessed 19.04.22).
[132] USDA; FDA. *Food and Agriculture: Considerations for Prioritization of PPE, Cloth Face Coverings, Disinfectants, and Sanitation Supplies During the COVID-19 Pandemic*. Available from: https://www.fda.gov/food/food-safety-during-emergencies/food-and-agriculture-considerations-prioritization-ppe-cloth-face-coverings-disinfectants-and; 2021 (accessed 19.04.22).
[133] WHO. *Cleaning and Disinfection of Environmental Surfaces in the Context of COVID-19*. Available from: https://www.who.int/publications/i/item/cleaning-and-disinfection-of-environmental-surfaces-inthe-context-of-covid-19; 2021 (accessed 19.04.22).
[134] FDA. *Best Practices for Re-Opening Retail Food Establishments during the COVID-19 Pandemic*. Available from: https://www.fda.gov/food/food-safety-during-emergencies/best-practices-re-opening-retail-food-establishments-duringcovid-19-pandemic; 2021 (accessed 19.04.22).
[135] The Food and Drug Administration (FDA) and the Occupational Safety and Health Administration (OSHA). *Employee Health and Food Safety Checklist for Human and Animal Food Operations During the COVID-19 Pandemic*. Available from: https://www.fda.gov/food/food-safety-during-emergencies/employee-health-and-food-safety-checklist-human-andanimal-food-operations-during-covid-19-pandemic; 2021 (accessed 19.04.22).

[136] CDC; FDA. *Protecting Seafood Processing Workers from COVID-19.* Available from: https://www.cdc.gov/coronavirus/2019-ncov/community/guidance-seafood-processing.html; 2021 (accessed 19.04.22).
[137] CDC. *Meat and Poultry Processing Workers and Employers.* Available from: https://www.cdc.gov/coronavirus/2019-ncov/community/organizations/meat-poultry-processing-workers-employers.html; 2019 (accessed 19.04.22).
[138] J. Zhang, X. Fang, Y. Mao, H. Qi, J. Wu, X. Liu, et al., Real-time, selective, and low-cost detection of trace level SARS-CoV-2 spike-protein for cold-chain food quarantine, NPJ Sci. Food 5 (1) (2021) 1−6.
[139] S. Riddell, S. Goldie, A. Hill, D. Eagles, T.W. Drew, The effect of temperature on persistence of SARS-CoV-2 on common surfaces, Virol. J. 17 (1) (2020) 1−7.

CHAPTER TWO

Fourier transform infrared spectroscopy combined with multivariate analysis for quality analysis of fats and oils

Abdul Rohman[1,2] and Gunawan Indrayanto[3]
[1]Center of Excellence, Institute for Halal Industry and System (IHIS), Gadjah Mada University, Yogyakarta, Indonesia
[2]Department of Pharmaceutical Chemistry, Faculty of Pharmacy, Gadjah Mada University, Yogyakarta, Indonesia
[3]Faculty of Pharmacy, Surabaya University, Surabaya, Indonesia

2.1 Introduction

Edible fats and oils are essential for daily human diet because they provide high energy, nutrients, essential fatty acids, and some minor components such as fat-soluble vitamins, phenolics, and carotenoids. In the last decades, the demand for edible fats and oils has increased, which has led to their large production rate [1]. For frying oils, palm oil is regarded as the most consumed oil, and the highest production of palm oil in the world is in Indonesia, and therefore, palm oil is indeed an export commodity. Besides, some oils mainly coming from marine are excellent sources of omega-3 and omega-6 essential fatty acids [2]. Certain edible fats and oils are also correlated with remarkable health benefits, such as reducing the risk of cardiovascular disease, working as antioxidant by blocking the oxidation reaction of polyunsaturated fatty acids induced by free radicals, and reducing the metabolic diseases [3].

Chemically, edible fats and oils are mainly composed of glycerol esterified with three fatty acids known as triacylglycerols (TAGs) with some minor components responsible for certain biological activities such as fat-soluble vitamins including tocopherols, carotenoids, and phenolic contents [4]. The physical and chemical properties affect the quality of fats and oils, and therefore, it is very important to evaluate these properties in detail. The refractive index, color, specific gravity, melting point, and viscosity

Food Quality Analysis.
DOI: https://doi.org/10.1016/B978-0-323-95988-9.00007-2

are among the parameters to be evaluated physically, while acid value (AV), saponification value (SV), iodine value (IV), fatty acid and TAG composition, unsaponifiable matters such as tocopherols and sterols as well as minor components such as chlorophyll pigments and phospholipids (PLs) are chemical properties which are typically evaluated for quality control of edible fats and oils [5].

Fats and oils are prone to oxidation reactions during storage and processing. The oxidation reaction is accelerated by the presence of high temperature, oxygen, light, and metal ions. During auto-oxidation, fats and oils are oxidized through free-radical chain reaction involving the steps of initiation, propagation, and termination to result in the primary of hydroperoxides (HPs) and secondary oxidation products. HPs are easily decomposed into some small compounds of alcohols, hydrocarbons, aldehydes, and ketones known as secondary oxidation products. The secondary oxidation products are volatile, which make off-flavors in edible fats oils less. Some parameters are used to evaluate the stability of fats and oils including polar compounds, peroxide value (PV), anisidine value (AnV), carbonyl value (CaV), and thiobarbituric acid reactive substances (TBARS) or thiobarbituric value (TBA-V) [6].

Some official methods appearing in American Oil Chemists' Society (AOCS), Japan Oil Chemists' Society (JOCS), the International Union of Pure and Applied Chemists (IUPAC), and Association of Official Analytical Chemists (AOAC) have been well documented for the evaluation of physical and chemical properties as well as the oxidation parameter quality control of fats and oils. Analysis of parameters of fats and oils is typically based on titrimetric or volumetric analyses, which involve the extensive use of solvents and reagents. Thus, some green analytical methods based on vibrational spectroscopy including infrared (IR) spectroscopy are widely developed, validated, and applied for these tasks [5,6]. The data generated during the scanning of Fourier transform infrared (FTIR) spectra are large even from the single measurement, and therefore, FTIR spectroscopic method is typically combined with multivariate data analysis or chemometrics.

2.2 Fourier transform infrared spectroscopy and chemometrics

For the last decade, FTIR spectroscopy has emerged as a powerful analytical technique in several fields such as food, agriculture, biomedical, clinical fields, and pharmaceutical products. IR spectroscopy is one of molecular spectroscopies in which the absorption of energy leads to several excited molecular vibrational and rotational states to provide FTIR spectra. Recently, owing to the developments in FTIR spectrometer instrumentation and computer software, this technique is widely applied in qualitative and quantitative analyses [7]. The main advantages of FTIR spectroscopy are its simplicity, rapid, good reproducibility, non-destructive method, minimal or without sample preparation needed, and providing confirmation, qualitative and quantitative analyses. The disadvantages of FTIR spectroscopy include the need to build a new calibration model if the sample composition is different, attenuated total reflectance (ATR) spectra need further processing to obtain the significance on a molecular level, and the selection of ATR crystal influence the resulted FTIR spectra [8,9].

The wavenumbers ($1/\lambda$) of IR regions are classified into three regions relative to ultraviolet−visible region, namely, near-IR ($1/\lambda$ 14,000−4000/cm), mid-IR ($1/\lambda$ 4000−400/cm), and far-IR region ($1/\lambda$ of 400−50/cm). Among these, the mid-IR is the most widely employed region for the monitoring of parameters of fats and oils as well as the most used technique for authentication analysis of fats and oils, followed by near-IR spectroscopy and far-IR spectroscopy [10]. The employment of FTIR spectra to quality control of edible fats and oils depends on the valuable chemical parameters obtained from spectra in the mid-IR region. Among FTIR spectra regions, peaks at wavenumbers of 1500−600/cm are known as the fingerprint spectral region, which can be exploited for the characterization and authentication of fats and oils. Bands or shoulders come from the absorption of IR beam by functional groups in edible fats. Each band was characterized by wavenumbers to which functional groups absorb, the peak intensity (strong, medium, weak), peak shapes (broad and sharp), and the type of vibrations (symmetric and asymmetric stretching vibration, bending) [11]. Edible fats and oils are mainly composed of TAGs (Fig. 2.1), and therefore, the functional groups of TAGs dominate FTIR spectra. The main functional groups present in FTIR spectra are carbonyl (C = O), methyl, and methylene groups, *cis* = CH, ester linkage, etc. [12]. Fig. 2.2 reveals the ATR-FTIR spectra of edible fats and oils along with the wavenumbers, which is specific for certain functional groups.

FTIR spectra provide large datasets (big data) even from a single scan, and therefore, the use of sophisticated statistical software with chemometrics is a must [11]. Chemometrics is a field that is related to the employment of statistics and mathematics to treat chemical data (peaks in FTIR spectra with

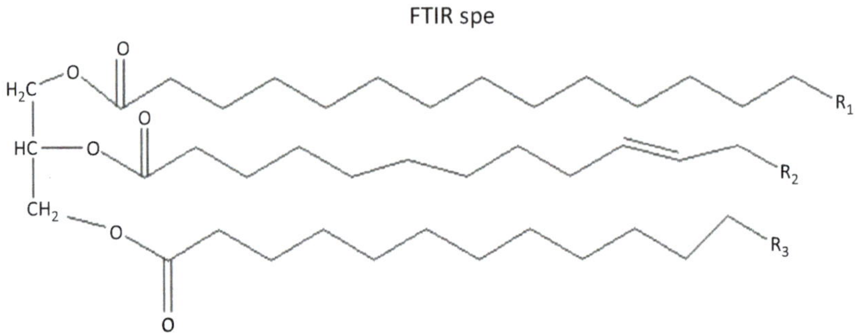

Figure 2.1 Triacylglycerol, three fatty acid esterified with glycerol, the main component in edible fats and oils [13].

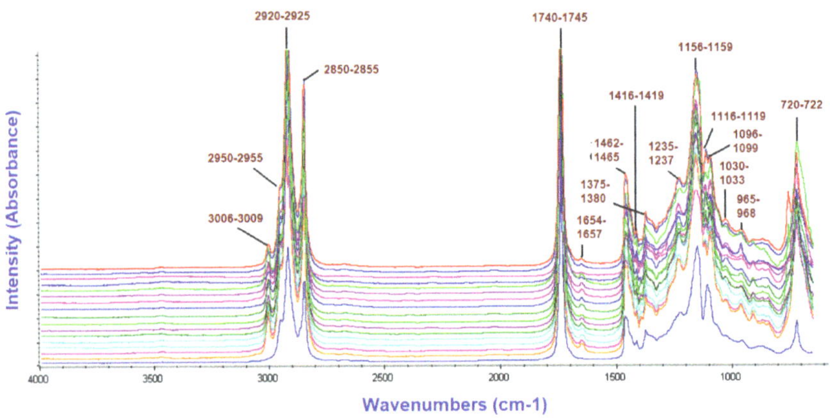

Figure 2.2 ATR-FTIR spectra of edible fats and oils in mid-IR region (4000–650/cm) along with the wavenumbers related to the functional groups absorbing infrared beam. Figure is taken from Rohman's dissertation (2010). ATR-FTIR, *Attenuated total reflectance-Fourier transform infrared spectroscopy*.

different wavenumbers and intensity). The International Chemometrics Society has defined chemometrics as the science that correlates the chemical measurements (chemical responses) made on a chemical system with the property of interest (such as concentration) through the application of mathematical or statistical methods [14]. The development of computer technology, software, and statistics has contributed to the wide application of chemometrics in several fields including biochemistry, food, agriculture, etc. Some user-friendly software are available either commercially or open sources such as Minitab, Unscrambler, R program for Statistics Computing, SIMCA, and MATLAB®PLS_Toolbox. Brereton et al. [15] reviewed the applicability of each chemometrics software [16]. In fats and oils studies, chemometric software are important for decision-making and problem-solving processes during differentiation of fats and oils and prediction of oil's parameters [17,18].

The most common chemometrics methods applied during the quality control of fats and oils are multivariate calibration, which correlate the actual values of fat and oil parameters as determined by means of official methods such as those published in AOAC, JOCS, or AOCS methods and predict values using the developed methods (FTIR spectroscopy). Stepwise multiple linear regression, principal component regression (PCR), and partial least square (PLS) are among multivariate calibrations used in fat and oil analyses. In addition, exploratory data analysis such as principal component analysis (PCA), unsupervised pattern recognition such as cluster analysis, and supervised pattern recognition including linear discriminant analysis and soft independent modeling by class analogy are also used for the classification and discrimination of fats and oils. The chemometrics of preprocessing spectra such as derivatization, smoothing, mean centering, and standard normal variate (SNV) are also widely used during the optimization of prediction modeling [6,19] (Table 2.1).

Table 2.1 The correlation between peak's wavenumbers and functional groups composed triacylglycerols [20,21].

Wavenumbers (cm^{-1})	Functional group	Mode of vibration	Intensity
3006–3009	$=C-H$ (*cis*)	Stretching	Medium
2950–2955	Methyl ($-CH_3$)	Asymmetric stretching	Medium
2920–2925	$-CH_2$ (methylene)	Asymmetric stretching	Very strong
2850–2855	$-CH$ (methylene)	Symmetric stretching	Very strong
1740–1745	$-C=O$ (ester)	Stretching	Very strong
1654–1657	$-C=C$ (*cis*)	Stretching	Very weak
1462–1466	$-CH_2$ (methylene)	Bending (scissoring)	Very weak
1416–1419 (b)	$=C-H$ (*cis*-disubstituted olefins)	Bending (rocking)	Weak
1375–1380	$-CH_3$ (methyl)	Bending (symmetric)	Medium
1235–1237	$-C-O$; $-CH_2-$	Stretching; bending	Medium
1156–1159	$-C-O$; $-CH_2-$	Stretching; bending	Strong
1116–1119	$-C-O$ (ether linkage)	Stretching	Medium
1096–1099	$-C-O$	Stretching	Medium
1030–1033	$-C-O$	Stretching	Very weak
965–968	$-HC=CH-$ (*trans*)	Out of plane	Weak
720–722	$-(CH_2)_n$; $-HC=CH-$ (*cis*)	Bending (rocking)	Medium

2.3 Analysis of fat and oil components

FTIR spectroscopy in combination with chemometric is an ideal technique for quantitative analysis of lipid components in fats and oils. Park et al. [22] validated FTIR spectroscopy for quantification of phosphatidylcholine (PC) and total PL in krill oil. The absorbance values of FTIR spectra corresponding to functional groups of choline and phosphate were optimized during determination of PC and total PL. The latter was characterized by peaks corresponding to asymmetric and symmetric stretching vibrations of phosphate diester PO_2- (1236 and 1090/cm), asymmetric and symmetric vibrations of ester stretch in $-C-O-P$ (1167 and 1060/cm), and asymmetric stretching vibration of $-N-(CH_3)_3$ at wavenumbers of 970/cm. The authors also compared the performance of FTIR normal spectra and the second derivative in terms of providing the best models (highest R^2 for accuracy and low errors). Finally, the second derivative FTIR spectra at wavenumbers of 970/cm corresponding to asymmetric stretching vibration of $(CH_3)_3-N$ was selected for quantitative analysis of PC. The correlation between actual values of PC as determined by $^{31}P-NMR$ method as specified in Codex (x-axis), and FTIR-predicted values (y-axis) provided an equation of $y = 0.00513 + 0.014$ with R^2 of 0.999, while PL was determined using the second derivative spectra at -1236/cm originating from $P = O$ asymmetric stretching signal having R^2-values of 0.998. Using this method, the values of limit of detection was found to be in the range of 0.35–3.29 with recoveries for accuracy evaluation of method of 97.90%–100.33%. The precision, expressed as relative standard deviations (RSD) for repeatability, was acceptable in the range of 0.90%–2.31%. These results were confirmed to be comparable with standard method for analysis of PC and PL, that is, ^{31}P NMR spectroscopy. Therefore, FTIR spectra could be alternative method for analysis of PL and PC in edible fats and oils.

FTIR spectra obtained from NaCl windows using transmission path fixed at 50 μm was applied for quantitative analysis of tert-butylhydroquinone (TBHQ), a synthetic antioxidant added in edible fats and oils, in palm olein samples. Absorbance values at 3600 and 2800 cm^{-1} were used for the prediction of TBHQ in the samples. In this study, 50 palm olein samples were spiked with known amounts of TBHQ up to 300 mg/kg (ppm) and then divided into calibration and validation datasets. Partial least squares regression (PLS-R) was used for establishing the correlation between actual values of TBHQ as determined using IUPAC based on HPLC method and FTIR-predicted values. R2 value-calibration of 0.9961, R2 value-validation of 0.9951, standard error of calibration (SEC) of 5.06, and standard error of prediction (SEP) of 6.49 were obtained during method validation. Furthermore, there no significant difference ($P < .05$) was observed for the accuracy and repeatability results between IUPAC method and FTIR spectroscopy, indicating that the developed method is suitable for the routine quality control of TBHQ in fats and oils [23].

2.4 Determination of fat and oil parameters using Fourier transform infrared spectroscopy

Fats and oils have been characterized by several parameters including thermal and oxidation stabilities. The oxidation stability of oils is one of the most important parameters during quality control of edible fats and oils because it determines its usefulness and its shelf life [24]. In food chemistry, various methods are used to determine the oxidative stability of oils, and the most reliable test is the storage test, but it is very time-consuming, and therefore, some methods have been applied for the evaluation of fat and oil stability such as determination of free fatty acids (acid value), peroxide value for the assessment of primary oxidation products, AnV to evaluate secondary oxidation products, and induction period (IP) [25]. IP can be defined as the time between the initial measurement and the time when the formation of oxidation products rapidly begins to increase. This time can be used to assess when edible fats and oils reach the oxidation level that is unsuitable for human consumption [26]. AOCS and AOAC have recommended a standard method for analysis of fats and oils mainly using titrimetric methods (acid value, peroxide value) and ultraviolet–visible spectroscopic methods (determination of conjugated dienes or K232 and trienes or K270). The titration method typically uses a large amount of highly toxic, carcinogenic, and environmentally unfriendly organic solvents, and therefore, greener analytical method based on FTIR spectroscopy has been continuously developed as an alternative method. Table 2.2 summarizes the reported applications of FTIR spectroscopy in combination with chemometrics for analysis of oil parameters.

Table 2.2 The application of FTIR (Fourier transform infrared spectroscopy) spectroscopy and chemometrics for the prediction of fats and oils parameters.

Fat and oil parameter	FTIR condition and chemometrics	Results	Ref.
Analysis of AVs of 105 samples from different oil samples	FTIR spectra at wavenumbers of 3340–3390/cm and PLS-R	The PLS-R model for the correlation between actual AV as determined by AOCS method provided R^2 value of 0.9921. The absolute deviation is less 0.2 AV. The AV of studied oils analyzed using FTIR spectra is in agreement with that analyzed using the AOCS method	[27]
Determination of PVs in fish oils	The combined region of 3816–2524 and 1800–828/cm	Using PLS-1 regression employing absorbance values at this region as variable, the correlation between actual values of TBARS and FTIR predicted values provided R^2 values of 0.967, SEC of 0.07, SECV of 0.110, RDP of 3.67, and bias of −0.0022	[28]
Analysis of TBARS values in palm oils	The combined regions at 2900–2800 and 1800–1600/cm	PLS-R provided the close relationship between actual values of TBARS and predicted value with R^2 values of 0.9803, the number of factors of 5, and SEC value of 0.0063–0.0680, and SEP of 1.20–6.67	[28]

(*Continued*)

Table 2.2 (Continued)

Fat and oil parameter	FTIR condition and chemometrics	Results	Ref.
Determination of TBARS values in the range of 0–60 μmol malonaldehyde/kg palm olein oils	The combined regions at 2900–2800 and 1800–1600/cm	PLS-R using variable of absorbance values at this region provided R^2 values of 0.9891 and SEC of 1.49 for the correlation between actual values of TBARS as determined by standard method and FTIR method. Cross-validation of calibration model provided R2 of 0.9786 and SEP of 2.136	[29]
Determination of TBARS in fish oils	The combined region of 3816–2524 and 1800–828/cm	Using PLS-1 regression, the correlation between actual values of TBARS and FTIR predicted values provided R^2 values of 0.969, SEC of 0.06, SECV of 0.136, RDP of 3.23, and bias of 0.004	
Determination of Ca-V in frying oils	FTIR spectra at wavenumbers of 4000–650/cm and PLS-R	FTIR spectra combined with PLS-R was successful for predicting the carbonyl value of frying oils. R^2 values, SECV, and SEP were 0.99, 1.87, and 1.93 μmol/g, respectively	[30]

SEC, standard error of calibration; *SEP*, standard error of prediction.

Owing to a large number of peaks and fingerprint property of the FTIR spectra, an analyst could determine the parameters of fats and oils simultaneously by selecting the specific peaks, which are directly correlated with these parameters. For example, free fatty acid value (FFAV) and AV could be related to functional groups related to COOH (large peak around 3400/cm), iodine value could be related to peaks originating from unsaturated functional groups such as *cis*-double bond of =CH– (around 3007/cm), while peroxide values and other oxidation products could be related to peroxide absorptions [6,21].

During thermal oxidation, there are some changes in FTIR spectra of edible fats and oils, in which the intensities of certain peaks are increased or decreased according to the addition or reduction of certain compounds [29]. For example, broad peak with low intensity appeared at 3473/cm corresponding to O–H stretching vibration of hydroperoxides, formed during the lipid peroxidation of polyunsaturated lipids. Inversely, the peak intensity at wavenumbers of 3008/cm due to stretching vibration of *cis* = C–H was decreased with the increased degree of fat and oil oxidation [30]. Selaimia et al. [31] also reported that during heating of olive oil at 90°C, there are some changes in peak intensities, namely, at spectral regions of 3480–2670/cm due to stretching vibrations of fatty acids and hydroperoxides and at 1750–720/cm due to conjugated bonds and of bending vibrations of aliphatic compounds. Lard (pork fat) subjected to high temperature of 300°C also revealed decreased intensity at 721/cm, implying the loss of *cis*-double bonds during oxidation. This fact was confirmed by the decreased intensity of peaks at 3006/cm, assigned to the same *cis*-double bonds C = CH [32]. Zahir et al. also reported peak intensities corresponding to carbonyl (C = O) stretching vibration at 1745.5 cm^{-1} and aliphatic C–H (methyl– and methylene–) at 2853–2926/cm in corn oil heated at 170°C [33]. This phenomenon could be exploited for making the relationship between the intensity changes of certain peaks in FTIR spectra with certain fat and oil parameters.

1. Analysis of AVs

   AVs are defined as the amount of potassium hydroxide (KOH) in milligrams required to neutralize FFAs in 1 g edible fats and oils. This value is represented by the amount of fatty acids present in fats and oils. Fatty acids are released during the processing or during the hydrolysis of fats and oils, and therefore, AVs could be used as an indication of fat and oil quality because FFAs are typically formed during decomposition of TAGs due to the action of moisture, temperature, and/or lipase enzymes. The official method for determination of AVs is acid–base titration in which fats and oils are directly titrated in neutral alcoholic solvent against standard KOH or NaOH. For example, the AOCS method for AV is Cd 3a-63.1, while AOCS Ca 5a-40 is used for analysis of FFAs. These methods involve organic solvents and reagents, which can contaminate the environment. Therefore, some alternative methods, for example, FTIR spectroscopy, have been proposed and developed for determination of AVs and FFAVs [27].

The combination of multivariate calibration and FTIR spectra using the characteristic peak due to stretching vibration of O–H attached to carboxyl groups in FFAs was developed as alternative method for determination of AVs in 105 samples of edible oils, namely, peanut, rapeseed, soybean, and palm oils. The PLS-R model for the correlation between actual AV as determined by AOCS method and FTIR spectra at wavenumbers of 3340–3390/cm provide R^2-value of 0.9921. Furthermore, the bias observed between actual value and FTIR-predicted value was low, in which 61 of 75 samples had the absolute deviation of less than 0.1 AV, and more than 95% of the oil samples (73 of 75 samples) had the absolute deviation less than 0.2 AV units regardless the types of studied fats and oils. This result indicated that the AV of studied oils analyzed using FTIR spectra is in agreement with that analyzed using the official method [34]. The other applications of FTIR spectra for determining AV are compiled in Table 2.2.

FTIR spectra obtained using spectral accessory method of infrared quartz cuvette (IQC) have been developed for prediction of AV of edible oils. PLS-R was used for constructing the calibration models between actual values of AVs as determined using titration method according to official method (OCS Cd 20–91) and FTIR-predicted values. The absorbance values of the first derivative spectra at region of 3603–3250/cm offered the best prediction models for AVs of edible oils (in this study, oils used are rapeseed, linseed, cottonseed, peanut, soybean, sesame, sunflower, walnut, *Silybum marianum* seed oils and their mixture). The equation used for prediction of AVs is: predicted AV values (y) = 0.9956 x actual values + 0.0008 (0.9968 and SD of 0.1343 AV). Validation using calibration samples and blind samples presented a good agreement of FTIR spectroscopy with official titrimetric methods. Thus, FTIR spectroscopy provides an alternative method for analysis of AVs in edible fats and oils [35].

2. Determination of peroxide values

FTIR spectroscopy was combined with two multivariate calibrations (PLS-R and PCR) for predicting PVs in virgin walnut oil (VWO) samples subjected to heating treatments. PLS-R using absorbance values at combined wavenumbers of 3009–1041/cm was exploited for the relationship between actual values of PVs as determined by official methods using titrimetric method (x-axis) and FTIR-predicted values providing R^2-values of 0.9918 and 0.9903 with standard deviations of 0.236 and 0.257 (in calibration and validation models). In addition, the precision of analytical method was acceptable as indicated by low root mean square errors of calibration (RMSEC) value of 0.4838 meq/kg and 0.3545 meq/kg, respectively. The developed method is a potential alternative technique for determining PVs of edible fats and oils [36]. FTIR spectroscopy can be used for simultaneous analysis of analytes (or oil parameters) by selecting the specific peaks corresponding to specific analytes. Based on this, Faridah et al. [37] presented FTIR spectroscopy and multivariate calibration of ordinary least square (OLS) for determining PVs and FFAVs of palm oils used to fry catfish. In this study, two batches of commercial PaO were used for frying catfish nine times at 180°C for 15 min. The used PaO were subjected to FTIR spectral measurement at wavenumbers of 4000–400/cm using KBr disk to form a KBr disk sandwich. FTIR spectra were then used to predict FFAVs and PVs, while the actual values of FFAVs and PVs were determined using official method of AOCS Ca 5a-40 and AOCS Cd 8–53, respectively. The correlation between actual values (x-axis) and FTIR-predicted values (y-axis) can be expressed by the equation:

$$\begin{aligned}\%\text{FFA value} = & -161.34 + 0.74xA_{722} + 7.02xA_{872} + 3.50xA_{912.5} \\ & + 1.11xA_{1091} + 2.30xA_{1130} + 1.44xA_{1400.5} \\ & + 1.49xA_{1418} + 1.01xA_{1.654} + 1.59xA_{729} + 1.9xA_{2974} \\ & + 1.09xA_{3005.54} + 4.25xA_{3474.91} - 2.14xA_{3530};\end{aligned}$$

where A_{722} is the absorbance value of PaO in wavenumbers 722 nm. The R2 values obtained were of 0.955 at *P* value .042 ($P < .05$) indicating that there is a significant correlation between actual values of percent FFA and absorbance values at selected wavenumbers used for prediction.

In addition, the predicted PVs are expressed as:

$$\begin{aligned}PV = & \, 3284.74 - 37.89xA_{722} + 136.08xA_{872} - 62.67xA_{912.5} \\ & -183.24xA_{966} - 17.61xA_{1091} - 32.70xA_{1130} \\ & -27.97xA_{1400.5} - 53.34xA_{1418} + 30.66xA_{1654} - 30.22xA_{1729} \\ & -40.09xA_{2974.36} - 33.56xA_{3005.54} - 111.92xA_{3474.91}\end{aligned}$$

The R^2 value of 0.963 with *P* value of .030 ($P < .05$). This result indicated that combination of FTIR spectroscopy and OLS can provide accurate and reliable method for simultaneous determination of

FFAVs and PVs without any sample preparation technique, and therefore, this method supports the campaign of green analytical method [19]. Recently, some improvements on multivariate calibrations of PLS-R using the calculation of PVs using ridge regression, LASSO regression, and elastic net regression model were reported, and these models provide better prediction of PVs [38].

3. Analysis of SV

The SV was expressed as the amount of KOH (in milligrams). This value is specific for certain oils and is inversely proportional with molecular weight of fats and oils. Fats and oils with low molecular weights exhibit high SVs, and therefore, SV is widely applied for characterization and authentication of high-quality fats and oils [39]. FTIR spectroscopy combined with the multivariate calibrations has been developed for prediction of SV in edible fats and oils. Putri et al. [28] used FTIR and PLS using optimum variable of absorbance values of the first derivative spectra at 1007–1600/cm for determination of PVs in patin fish oils extracted from different extraction methods using different extracting solvents. PLS method gave R^2-calibration and R^2-validation of 0.9970 and 0.999, respectively, with the RMSEC and root mean square error of prediction (RMSEP) were 4.54 and 4.45, respectively. A similar approach was also reported by Rohman et al., who used FTIR spectra for rapid analysis of SV in red fruit oil, and FTIR spectroscopy combined with multivariate calibrations provide the comparable results with those using reference methods (titrimetric methods) [40]. The other uses of FTIR spectra and multivariate calibrations are compiled in Table 2.2.

Our group have analyzed determined AVs, SV, and PV in patin fish oils extracted using maceration and Soxhlet by different solvents, namely, hexane, chloroform, and ethyl acetate. FTIR spectra modes and multivariate calibrations were optimized and compared to get the best prediction models using FTIR spectra. AVs of patin fish oils were best predicted using PCR applying the absorbance values at 3100–2000/cm as variables during modeling to provide R^2-cal, R^2-val, RMSEC, and RMSEP of 0.9983, 0.9999, 0.21, and 0.97, respectively. PLS using the first derivative FTIR spectra at 2111–1500/cm was suitable for determination of PVs, while SVs was predicted using PLS applying the first derivative spectra 1600–1007/cm with acceptable accuracy and precision as indicated by high R^2 and low RMSEC and RMSEP values [28].

4. Determination of IVs

IV is one of the great interest parameters in edible fats and oils for measuring the degree of unsaturation quickly. The functional groups related to the unsaturated functional groups (e.g., *cis*-double bonds or $=C-H$) can be target of analysis during the development of IR spectroscopy for prediction of IV. Besides, some analysts applied peak intensities related to stretching vibration of $C=C$ and scissoring vibration of CH_2 for the determination of total unsaturation degree [41]. Some other regions were also used for IV determination, as cited by Dymińska et al., namely, at the combined wavenumber of 2600–3200 and 1000–1600/cm or at combined regions of 1626–1691 and 1420–1478/cm or at wavenumbers of 1656–1444/cm, and at region of 3010–1270/cm [42]. The IVs are specific for certain fats and oils, and therefore, it can be used for early detection of edible fats and oils from potential adulterants. IV is defined as the amount of iodine (in grams) absorbed by 100 g edible fats and oils. The higher the IV, the more unsaturated fatty acid parts are present in fats and oils. The standard method for determination of IV as appeared in AOAC, AOCS, and JOCS involves the highly toxic reagents and solvents, which are environmentally unfriendly. Thus, FTIR spectroscopy in combination with chemometrics has the potential to be proposed as an alternative method for IV determination [43]. With the development of handheld vibrational spectrometers such as Fourier transform near infrared, Fourier transform mid infrared, and Raman spectrometer, it is possible to perform onsite determination of IV in edible fats and oils with rapidity and accuracy benefits [44].

Yan et al. [41] performed FTIR spectroscopy in combination with PLS and variable selection for determining IV in selected edible oils (soybean, olive, and peanut oils) along with their blends to get variety of IVs. The standard method based on ISO 3961:1996 procedure was used for determination of IV, and the results obtained were used as actual values to be correlated with predicted values of IV modeled using FTIR spectra in combination with PLS-R. Some improvements have been made in the developed method in which some variables (absorbance values in FTIR spectra) capable of providing the best model were selected using the chemometrics of Monte Carlo uninformative variables elimination, competitive reweighted sampling (CARS), bootstrapping soft shrinkage approach (BOSS) and variable combination population analysis. Then, the values of PLS and

RMSEP were used as indicative parameters for the predictability of PLS-R models. The results of PLS-R calibration models using FTIR spectra as variables were previously treated by CARS, SCARS, BOSS, and SBOSS. Before PLS-R modeling, FTIR spectra are mean-centered, and the optimal number of latent variables was determined by fivefold cross validation. RMSEC, RMSEP, Qcv^2, and $Qtest^2$ were used to evaluate model performance. FTIR spectra treated by CARS showed the best performance of prediction model with RMSEP value of 2.2185, RMSEC of 1.8038, Qcv^2 of 0.9724, and $Qtest^2$ of 0.9313. The reason that CARS provided a better model than other variable selections may be that variables are heavily collinear, and therefore, the variance of PLS-R model could be reduced with fewer variables.

5. Determination of thiobarbituric acid value

The secondary oxidation products were evaluated by determining TBARS, which is also known as "thiobarbituric acid value" (TBA-V). This value is typically used as a marker for secondary lipid peroxidation in fried fast foods and in the encapsulated products containing edible fats and oils [45]. Determination of TBA-V involved the reaction of malonaldehyde (MDA), as a representative of secondary oxidation product, with TBA in the medium of glacial acetic acid to yield a red-colored solution having maximum absorbance at 532 nm [46]. Mirghani et al. [47] evaluated the possibility of FTIR spectra in combination with two multivariate calibrations of PLS-R and PCR for prediction of TBARS in palm oil samples. The actual values of TBARS were evaluated by official method of AOCS method Cd 19–90, and some wavenumber regions were evaluated to provide the best prediction models. Finally, the combined regions at 2900–2800 and 1800–1600/cm corresponding to stretching vibrations –CH aldehyde and carbonyl were selected. During secondary oxidation process, aldehyde, ketone, hydrocarbon, alcohol, and ester with low molecular weights were formed, and therefore, it is appropriate to use these wavenumber regions. In this study, 50 samples of palm oil with TBA-Vs of 0–0.25 were used to build the calibration models based on PLS-R and PCR. PLS-R offer better TBA-V modeling than PCR with R^2 values of 0.9803, the number of factors of 5, and SEC value of 0.0063 to 0.0680, and SEP of 1.20 to 6.67. The values of RSD obtained using PLS-R was also lower than those using PCR. Therefore, FTIR spectra combined with PLS-R could be used as accurate (high R^2) and precise (low error) method for determining TBARS to assess the secondary oxidation products. Oleszko et al. [48] also determined TBARS using ATR-FTIR spectra, and there is a good correlation between TBARS and the absorbance ratios of carbonyl peaks (C = O) with CH_3 providing R^2 values of 0.991.

Determination of AVs, PVs, and TBA-Vs in palm oil (PaO) heated at 180°C for 72 hour h was also carried out using FTIR spectroscopy and multivariate calibration of PLS-OLS model. Some absorbance values in certain peaks of FTIR spectra (721.4, 871.8, 968.3, 1033.9, 1095.6, 1377.2, 1462, 1751.4, 2731.2, 2839.2, and 3005.1/cm) were optimized for making a reliable prediction of AVs, PVs, and TBA-Vs). The correlation between the actual values of AVs, PVs, TBA-Vs with FTIR-predicted values facilitated by PLS-OLS provided satisfactorily models with R^2 of 0.962, 0.857, and 0.845, respectively. The use of absorbance values at these wavenumbers provided significant effects to prediction of AVs, PVs, and TBA-Vs with *P*-values of $<.01$ [49].

6. Determination of total polar compounds

The studies related to the presence of total polar compounds (TPCs) in edible fats and oils, especially in frying oils, are widely reported because polar compounds have some health and nutritional implications. Therefore, some countries have limited the maximum levels of TPCs in edible oils. The main compositions of polar compounds include TAG oligomers, TAG dimers, oxidized TAG monomers, diglyceride and monoglycerides, as well as FFAs [50]. These TPCs increase linearly with the increased frying time. The common methods used for analysis of TPCs are silica gel column chromatography. Unfortunately, this method is time-consuming, tedious, and expensive. To overcome this obstacle, an alternative method using IR spectroscopy was proposed and validated [51].

Normally, the first and second derivative spectra at wavenumbers of 4000–650/cm coupled with PLS-R were compared for the prediction of TPCs in frying oils. The actual values of TPC were obtained from the direct measurement a food oil monitor based on the changes in dielectric constant. The results revealed that the first and second derivative spectra provide better performance with comparable accuracy than normal spectra. This can be explained that spectral derivatization could remove the baseline offset providing better prediction modeling [52]. Using six factors, PLS-R using the first derivative spectra exhibited a close relationship between actual values and FTIR-predicted values with R^2-calibration and R^2-validation of 0.98 with RMSEC of 1.05, root mean square error of cross-validation (RMSECV) of 1.17, and RMSEP of 1.10, bias of −0.10, and relative percent difference (RPD) of 7.3%. Bias is the average of differences between actual value and FTIR value, while RPD is ratio of standard deviation of actual value in the validation set to RMSEP. The wavenumbers contributing to the accurate prediction of TPC as evaluated from regression coefficients of the PLS is 3010, 2924, 2852, and 1716/cm, respectively [53]. FTIR spectroscopy combined with PLS-R was successfully applied to predict TPC in frying rapeseed oils with the precise and accurate prediction.

Furthermore, PVs, FFAVs, and IVs were also simultaneously predicted using FTIR and chemometrics. The spectra were subjected to preprocessing of SNV, MSC, and area normalization, followed by exploratory data analysis of PCA to identify the peaks (functional groups) providing the high load on the prediction. PLS-R was used to construct the relationship between these actual values and FTIR-predicted values of PVs, FFAVs, and IVs. The results showed that PLS-R using FTIR spectra subjected to normalization gave better results with R^2 values of calibration of 0.99 and 0.98 and R^2 of cross-validation of 0.84, 0.76, and 0.85 for PVs, FFAVs, and IVs, respectively. In addition, RMSEC and RMSECV obtained were in the range of 0.04−1.55 and 0.17−2.78, respectively. The developed method was applicable to predict FFAV (0.37%−1.63%), PV (4.47−13.85 meqO2/kg), and IV (111.51−51.39 I2/100 g) [54]. This result supports the application of FTIR spectroscopy as an effective technique for determination of fats and oils simultaneously.

7. Analysis of carbonyl value

Another oil parameter predicted using FTIR spectra and multivariate calibration of PLS-R is CaV in frying oils of rapeseed oil used for frying potato. During this study, 200 mL of heated oil was taken every 3.5 h, and CaV was determined using official method of the JOCS Method Tentative 13−2003 for determination of CaO. The results obtained was used as the actual value. The FTIR spectra mode (normal, derivatives) and the number of factors, a linear combination from original variable of absorbance values at certain wavenumbers, were optimized to get PLS-R model with the highest accuracy and lowest errors. Based on this optimization, the second derivative spectra with five factors was chosen for predicting CaV due to its capability to provide highest R^2 value in calibration and prediction of 0.98 and 0.97, respectively, with bias of −0.15, for the correlation between actual values of CaV and FTIR-predicted values. The error values were expressed as SEC of 1.68, SECV of 1.87, SEP of 1.93, and RPD of 5.8%. Based on the regression coefficients of the PLS-R, the peaks at wavenumbers of 3026, 3008, 1736, 1147, and 968/cm were more contributing toward the prediction of CaV. This is not surprising that the peak intensity at 1736/cm related to the absorption of carbonyl group (C = O) associated with aldehyde and ketone is increased as the content of carbonyl was increased during the more extensive degradation of frying oils [55]. This result confirmed that CaV of frying oils can be successfully predicted using the combination of FTIR spectra and PLS-R.

FTIR spectroscopy using sampling technique of polyethylene-film-based in combination with PLSR was applied for predicting IP of walnut oil (WO) [56]. Officially, IP was determined according to the methods of the American Oil Chemists Society named by AOCS Cd 12c-16 (accelerated oxidation test for the determination of the oxidation stability of fats and oils) known as Oxitest. The results obtained using Oxitest method is referred to as the actual values of IP. The value of IP represents the oxidation stability of WO. During this study, the peak intensities at wavenumbers of 3008, 1654, 914, and 723/cm changed significantly as the IP value decreased, and this spectral intensity change could be used for the prediction of IP value. After the optimization step, the normal FTIR spectra at wavenumbers of 1640−440/cm were used for predicting IP values. Using this condition, the plots correlating between actual values of IP as determined using Oxitest and FTIR-predicted values provided R^2 value of 0.9847 and RMSEC of 3.38 (in calibration model), and R^2 value of 0.9878 and RMSEP of 2.32 (in validation model). The developed method was used for analysis of blind samples, and the obtained values R^2 and RMSEV were 0.9948% and 3.61%, respectively. The present study confirmed that polyethylene-FTIR method in combination of IP was suitable for analyzing the IP value of WO offering simple and rapid method for authentication analysis of WO.

References

[1] N. Zhang, et al., "Analytical methods for determining the peroxide value of edible oils: a mini-review, Food Chem. 358 (April) (2021) 129834. Available from: https://doi.org/10.1016/j.foodchem.2021.129834.

[2] A. Rohman, A.R. Putri, A. Irnawati, et al., The employment of analytical techniques and chemometrics for authentication of fish oils: a review, Food Control. 124 (2021). Available from: https://doi.org/10.1016/j.foodcont.2021.107864. vol.

[3] Y. Yao, B. Xu, New insights into chemical compositions and health promoting effects of edible oils from new resources, Food Chem. 364 (February) (2021) 130363. Available from: https://doi.org/10.1016/j.foodchem.2021.130363.

[4] X. Li, et al., Review of NIR spectroscopy methods for nondestructive quality analysis of oilseeds and edible oils, Trends Food Sci. Technol. 101 (May) (2020) 172–181. Available from: https://doi.org/10.1016/j.tifs.2020.05.002.

[5] Y. Endo, Analytical methods to evaluate the quality of edible fats and oils: the JOCS standard methods for analysis of fats, oils and related materials (2013) and advanced methods, J. Oleo Sci. 67 (1) (2018) 1–10. Available from: https://doi.org/10.5650/jos.ess17130.

[6] A. Rohman, Infrared spectroscopy for quantitative analysis and oil parameters of olive oil and virgin coconut oil: a review, Int. J. Food Prop. 20 (7) (2017) 1447–1456. Available from: https://doi.org/10.1080/10942912.2016.1213742.

[7] K.M. Fahelelbom, A. Saleh, M.M.A. Al-Tabakha, A.A. Ashames, Recent applications of quantitative analytical FTIR spectroscopy in pharmaceutical, biomedical, and clinical fields: a brief review, Rev. Anal. Chem. 41 (1) (2022) 21–33. Available from: https://doi.org/10.1515/revac-2022-0030.

[8] T. Sook Ling, S.H. Meriam Suhaimy, N.A. Abd Samad, Evaluation of fresh palm oil adulteration with recycled cooking oil using GC-MS and ATR-FTIR spectroscopy: a review, Czech J. Food Sci. 40 (1) (2022) 1–14. Available from: https://doi.org/10.17221/116/2021-cjfs.

[9] A. Rohman, Y.B. Che Man, Analysis of pig derivatives for halal authentication studies, Food Rev. Int. 28 (1) (2012) 97–112. Available from: https://doi.org/10.1080/87559129.2011.595862.

[10] R. Deidda, et al., Vibrational spectroscopy in analysis of pharmaceuticals: critical review of innovative portable and handheld NIR and Raman spectrophotometers, Trends Anal. Chem. 114 (2019) 251–259. Available from: https://doi.org/10.1016/j.trac.2019.02.035.

[11] R. Jamwal, et al., Recent trends in the use of FTIR spectroscopy integrated with chemometrics for the detection of edible oil adulteration, Vib. Spectrosc. 113 (January) (2021) 103222. Available from: https://doi.org/10.1016/j.vibspec.2021.103222.

[12] T.S.T. Mansor, Y.B.C. Man, A. Rohman, Application of fast gas chromatography and Fourier transform infrared spectroscopy for analysis of lard adulteration in virgin coconut oil, Food Anal. Methods 4 (3) (2011). Available from: https://doi.org/10.1007/s12161-010-9176-y.

[13] L. Andina, R. Saputri, A.N. Putri, A. Rohman, Infrared spectroscopy and multivariate calibration for the rapid quantification of free fatty acid content in pangasius hypopthalmus oil, Int. J. Appl. Pharm. 10 (6) (2018) 199–203. Available from: https://doi.org/10.22159/ijap.2018v10i6.28969.

[14] J.N. Miller, J.C. Miller, *Statistics and Chemometrics for Analytical* Chemistry, 6. ed, Prentice Hall, Harlow, 2010.

[15] R.G. Brereton, J. Jansen, J. Lopes, F. Marini, A. Pomerantsev, O. Rodionova, Chemometrics in analytical chemistry—part II: modeling, validation, and applications, Anal. Bioanal. Chem. 410 (2018) 6691–6704.

[16] I. Irnawati, F. Dika, O. Riswanto, S. Riyanto, S. Martono, The use of software package of R factoextra and FactoMineR and its application in principal componenet analysis for authentication of oils, Indones. J. Chemom. Pharm. Anal. 1 (1) (2021) 1–10.

[17] A.A. Christy, S. Kasemsumran, Y. Du, Y. Ozaki, The detection and quantification of adulteration in olive oil by near-infrared spectroscopy and chemometrics, Anal. Sci. 20 (6) (2004) 935–940. Available from: https://doi.org/10.2116/analsci.20.935.
[18] N. Hassan, T. Ahmad, N.M. Zain, Chemical and chemometric methods for halal authentication of gelatin: an overview, J. Food Sci. 83 (12) (2018) 2903–2911. Available from: https://doi.org/10.1111/1750-3841.14370.
[19] J. Moros, S. Garrigues, M. de la Guardia, Vibrational spectroscopy provides a green tool for multi-component analysis, Trends Anal. Chem. 29 (7) (2010) 578–591. Available from: https://doi.org/10.1016/j.trac.2009.12.012.
[20] M.J. Lerma-García, G. Ramis-Ramos, J.M. Herrero-Martínez, E.F. Simó-Alfonso, Authentication of extra virgin olive oils by Fourier-transform infrared spectroscopy, Food Chem. 118 (1) (2010) 78–83. Available from: https://doi.org/10.1016/j.foodchem.2009.04.092.
[21] A. Rohman, A. Nugroho, E. Lukitaningsih, Sudjadi, Application of vibrational spectroscopy in combination with chemometrics techniques for authentication of herbal medicine, Appl. Spectrosc. Rev. 49 (8) (2014) 603–613. Available from: https://doi.org/10.1080/05704928.2014.882347.
[22] S.E. Park, H.Y. Yu, S. Ahn, Development and validation of a simple method to quantify contents of phospholipids in krill oil by fourier-transform infrared spectroscopy, Foods 11 (1) (2022). Available from: https://doi.org/10.3390/foods11010041.
[23] W. Ammawath, Y.B.C. Man, B.S. Baharin, R.B.A. Rahman, A new method for determination of tert-butylhydroquinone (TBHQ) in RBD palm olein with FTIR spectroscopy, J. Food Lipids 11 (4) (2004) 266–277. Available from: https://doi.org/10.1111/j.1745-4522.2004.01142.x.
[24] Q. Li, et al., Application of Fourier transform infrared spectroscopy for the quality and safety analysis of fats and oils: a review, Critical Reviews in Food Science and Nutrition 59 (22) (2019) 3597–3611. Available from: https://doi.org/10.1080/10408398.2018.1500441.
[25] M. Maszewska, A. Florowska, E. Dłuzewska, M. Wroniak, K. Marciniak-Lukasiak, A. Zbikowska, Oxidative stability of selected edible oils, Molecules 23 (7) (2018) 15–17. Available from: https://doi.org/10.3390/molecules23071746.
[26] R. Hu, T. He, Z. Zhang, Y. Yang, M. Liu, Safety analysis of edible oil products via Raman spectroscopy, Talanta 191 (2019) 324–332. Available from: https://doi.org/10.1016/j.talanta.2018.08.074 (May 2018).
[27] A. Rohman, The use of infrared spectroscopy in combination with chemometrics for quality control and authentication of edible fats and oils: a review, Appl. Spectrosc. Rev. 52 (7) (2017) 589–604. Available from: https://doi.org/10.1080/05704928.2016.1266493.
[28] A.R. Putri, A. Rohman, W. Setyaningsih, S. Riyanto, Determination of acid, peroxide, and saponification value in patin fish oil by ftir spectroscopy combined with chemometrics, Food Res. 4 (5) (2020) 1758–1766. Available from: https://doi.org/10.26656/fr.2017.4(5).030.
[29] A. Rohman, Y.B. Che Man, Application of FTIR spectroscopy for monitoring the stabilities of selected vegetable oils during thermal oxidation, Int. J. Food Prop. 16 (7) (2013). Available from: https://doi.org/10.1080/10942912.2011.603874.
[30] Y. Lu, C. Du, Y. Shao, J. Zhou, Characterization of rapeseed oil using FTIR-ATR spectroscopy, J. Food Sci. Eng. 4 (May) (2014) 244–249. Available from: https://doi.org/10.17265/2159-5828/2014.05.004.
[31] R. Selaimia, R. Oumeddour, S. Nigri, The chemometrics approach applied to FTIR spectral data for the oxidation study of Algerian extra virgin olive oil, Int. Food Res. J. 24 (3) (2017) 1301–1307.

[32] A.A. Bunaciu, S. Fleschin, H.Y. Aboul-Enein, FTIR spectroscopy used for study the thermal degradation of lard, Egypt. Pharm. J. 20 (2) (2021) 166–172. Available from: https://doi.org/10.4103/0003-2778.320252.
[33] E. Zahir, R. Saeed, M.A. Hameed, A. Yousuf, Study of physicochemical properties of edible oil and evaluation of frying oil quality by Fourier Transform-Infrared (FT-IR) Spectroscopy, Arab. J. Chem. 10 (2017) S3870–S3876. Available from: https://doi.org/10.1016/j.arabjc.2014.05.025. vol.
[34] X. Jiang, et al., Determination of the acid values of edible oils via FTIR spectroscopy based on the O-H stretching band, Food Chem. 212 (2016) 585–589. Available from: https://doi.org/10.1016/j.foodchem.2016.06.035. vol.
[35] K. Hu, Z. Huyan, Q. Geng, X. Yu, Rapid determination of acid value of edible oils via ftir spectroscopy using inFrared Quartz Cuvette, J. Oleo Sci. 68 (2) (2019) 121–129. Available from: https://doi.org/10.5650/jos.ess18156.
[36] P. Liang, et al., Application of fourier transform infrared spectroscopy for the oxidation and peroxide value evaluation in virgin walnut oil, J. Spectrosc. 1 (1) (2013). Available from: https://doi.org/10.1155/2013/138728.
[37] D.N. Faridah, H.N. Lioe, N.S. Palupi, J. Kahfi, Detection of FFA and PV values using FTIR for quality measurement in palm oil frying activities, J. Oil Palm. Res. 27 (2) (2015) 156–167.
[38] W.E. Gilbraith, J.C. Carter, K.L. Adams, K.S. Booksh, J.M. Ottaway, Improving prediction of peroxide value of edible oils using regularized regression models, Molecules 26 (23) (2021). Available from: https://doi.org/10.3390/molecules26237281.
[39] C.A. Nunes, Vibrational spectroscopy and chemometrics to assess authenticity, adulteration and intrinsic quality parameters of edible oils and fats, Food Res. Int. 60 (2014) 255–261. Available from: https://doi.org/10.1016/j.foodres.2013.08.041. vol.
[40] A. Rohman, L. Triyasmono, S. Riyanto, L. Andina, Rapid determination of saponification value in red fruit oil by infrared spectroscopy and partial least square calibration, Res. J. Med. Plant. 9 (8) (2015). Available from: https://doi.org/10.3923/rjmp.2015.442.448.
[41] H. Yan, J. Zhang, J. Gao, Y. Huang, Y. Xiong, S. Min, Towards improvement in prediction of iodine value in edible oil system based on chemometric analysis of portable vibrational spectroscopic data, Sci. Rep. 8 (1) (2018) 1–9. Available from: https://doi.org/10.1038/s41598-018-33022-9.
[42] L. Dymińska, et al., Quantitative determination of the iodine values of unsaturated plant oils using infrared and Raman spectroscopy methods, Int. J. Food Prop. 20 (9) (2017) 2003–2015. Available from: https://doi.org/10.1080/10942912.2016.1230744.
[43] T. Kruatian, K. Jitmanee, Greener analytical method for determination of iodine number of edible oils, J. Food Res. 9 (6) (2020) 36. Available from: https://doi.org/10.5539/jfr.v9n6p36.
[44] S. Pulassery, B. Abraham, N. Ajikumar, A. Munnilath, K. Yoosaf, Rapid iodine value estimation using a handheld raman spectrometer for on-site, reagent-free authentication of edible oils, ACS Omega (2022). Available from: https://doi.org/10.1021/acsomega.1c05123.
[45] Z. Hu, Q. Zhong, Determination of thiobarbituric acid reactive substances in microencapsulated products, Food Chem. 123 (3) (2010) 794–799. Available from: https://doi.org/10.1016/J.FOODCHEM.2010.05.012.
[46] A. Zeb, F. Ullah, A simple spectrophotometric method for the determination of thiobarbituric acid reactive substances in fried fast foods, J. Anal. Methods Chem. 2016 (2016) 9412767. Available from: https://doi.org/10.1155/2016/9412767. vol.
[47] M.E.S. Mirghani, Y.B. Che Man, S. Jinap, B.S. Baharin, J. Bakar, Multivariate calibration of Fourier transform infrared spectra for determining thiobarbituric acid-

reactive substance content in palm oil, J. Am. Oil Chem. Soc. 78 (11) (2001) 1127–1131. Available from: https://doi.org/10.1007/s11746-001-0400-2.
[48] A. Oleszko, et al., Application of FTIR-ATR spectroscopy to determine the extent of lipid peroxidation in plasma during haemodialysis, Biomed. Res. Int. 2015 (2015) 1–9. Available from: https://doi.org/10.1155/2015/245607. vol.
[49] F. Kusnandar, H.N. Liou, D.N. Faridah, R. Anggraeni, P. Pricilia, Prediction of acid, peroxide and Tba values of heat-treated palm oil using a partial least squares–ordinary least squares model based on Fourier transform infrared spectroscopy, J. Oil Palm. Res. 33 (September) (2020) 514–523. Available from: https://doi.org/10.21894/jopr.2020.0106.
[50] X. Li, et al., Influence of fried food and oil type on the distribution of polar compounds in discarded oil during restaurant deep frying, Food Chem. 272 (2019) 12–17. Available from: https://doi.org/10.1016/j.foodchem.2018.08.023. no. August 2018.
[51] L. Xu, et al., Kinetics of forming polar compounds in frying oils under frying practice of fast food restaurants, Lwt 115 (2019). Available from: https://doi.org/10.1016/j.lwt.2019.108307. no. March.
[52] Å. Rinnan, F. van den Berg, S.B. Engelsen, Review of the most common preprocessing techniques for near-infrared spectra, Trends Anal. Chem. 28 (10) (2009) 1201–1222. Available from: https://doi.org/10.1016/j.trac.2009.07.007.
[53] J.Y. Chen, H. Zhang, J. Ma, T. Tuchiya, Y. Miao, Determination of the degree of degradation of frying rapeseed oil using fourier-transform infrared spectroscopy combined with partial least-squares regression, Int. J. Anal. Chem. 2015 (2015). Available from: https://doi.org/10.1155/2015/185367. vol.
[54] M.H. Ahmad, et al., Monitoring of frying process in canola oil blend using Fourier transform infrared and chemometrics techniques, Food Sci. Nutr. 9 (11) (2021) 6089–6098. Available from: https://doi.org/10.1002/fsn3.2558.
[55] A. Rohman, Y.B. Che Man, A. Ismail, P. Hashim, Monitoring the oxidative stability of virgin coconut oil during oven test using chemical indexes and FTIR spectroscopy, Int. Food Res. J. 18 (1) (2011) 303–310.
[56] Y. Wen, S. Zhou, L. Wang, Q. Li, Y. Gao, X. Yu, New method for the determination of the induction period of walnut oil by Fourier transform infrared spectroscopy, Food Anal. Methods 15 (3) (2022) 833–843. Available from: https://doi.org/10.1007/s12161-021-02170-6.

CHAPTER THREE

Fluorescence spectroscopy for beer quality analysis

Vivek Kumar and Arunima Singh
Department of Food Technology, Harcourt Butler Technical University, Kanpur, Uttar Pradesh, India

3.1 Introduction

Beer is a prominent and extensively used fermented alcoholic beverage produced from barley in the malted form. Hops are added to it for a stringent taste, and yeast along with water is added, and it is made by fermentation of sugary wort by immersing starch from different sources primarily malted barley in hot water, giving it a refreshing and pleasant taste [1]. Beer consists of a lot of healthy components like polyphenols, vitamin B, and minerals, which have a beneficial impact on healthy adults by reducing the chances of cardiovascular diseases, diabetes, and various types of cancers. Beer is composed of a variegated mixture of a number of ingredients differing widely in nature as well as concentration levels [2]. The raw materials like hops, yeast, and malt contain an extensive range of distinctive chemical components that react and interact with water at all the steps of the brewing process. There are various parameters like ingredients, storage conditions, and production processes that affect the characteristics of beer, and it is very important to analyze these conditions for estimating its organoleptic quality, nutritive value, and other quality and safety aspects [3]. It is known that no single compound is responsible for flavor, color, or other nutritional properties; rather, a very complex association of many diverse compounds is responsible for beer characteristics, and their presence or absence will lead to a unique flavor and taste. Thus, the analyses of all these compounds are essential to maintain uniform quality of beer throughout the process till consumption. Various analytical and chemical methods are mostly set up to quantify and characterize several properties of beer and its constituents. Likewise, photometry is used to determine bitterness and color, enzymatic methods or liquid

Food Quality Analysis.
DOI: https://doi.org/10.1016/B978-0-323-95988-9.00006-0

chromatography is used to determine organic acids, many volatile compounds and higher alcohols are detected by using gas chromatography [4]. However, pretreatment of samples is usually required in various analytical methods to set apart the targeted compounds in the concentrated form. These methods are time-intensive, costly, implicate the interference of unwanted organic solvents, and they require trained laboratory personnel. During the separation and fractionation process, the nature of the sample may get altered and lead to the retardation or dilution of various components.

The development of fast analytical methods that can be directly used for analyzing beer components and making extensive sample pretreatment unnecessary is of great interest for beverages and food analysis. Spectroscopic techniques facilitate very fast and noninvasive characterization of the samples and are especially fruitful in these applications. Spectroscopy techniques have the ability to analyze many compounds in single measurement rather than a single compound as in conventional methods. Practically, spectroscopic techniques are nondestructive, and measurements can be carried out very accurately in a simple manner, which makes it an intriguing method for sample characterization. Fluorescence spectroscopy is an alluring phenomenon owing to its increased responsivity to a wide array of potential analytes and selectivity compared to other absorption techniques, and its successful application in food analysis encourages its use for beer characterization [4]. Fluorescence is characterized under photoluminescence, a process in which a molecule is advanced to an electronically excited singlet state by absorbing near-infrared, ultraviolet (UV), or visible (Vis) radiation and declines back to its ground state by emanating a photon. The fluorescent analysis is beneficial due to the existence of natural fluorescent components of food or its contaminants. Fluorescence can also be added in food by accruing fluorophores or by making special derivatives of the analytes of the fluorescent compounds.

Conventional techniques of fluorescence rely on the analysis of single excitation or emission spectra and are generally insufficient in directly analyzing the complex systems. Multidimensional fluorescence techniques, such as synchronous fluorescence spectroscopy (SFS) and total luminescence spectroscopy (TLS) are specifically useful for analyzing complex food matrices. It gives the complete scanned intensity profile of excitation and emission wavelengths of the sample [5]. Synchronous fluorescence spectroscopy has advantages to scan both excitation and emission wavelength and analyze the difference in both the phenomenon [6]. Front-face fluorescence spectroscopy is also an innovative technique for food quality evaluation [7].

Fluorescence spectroscopy was used in many food products for determination of oxidation in fish and meat, and for the assay of milk, cheeses, and edible oils [8,9]. Apperson et al. [10] determined the fluorescence spectral data in different samples of diluted beer. Multivariate data analysis of autofluorescence spectrum of beer was used for evaluation of bitterness in beer [11]. A precise and sensitive fluorometric method was developed for estimating riboflavin content in beer [12]. TFS and SFS were used for differentiation of beer samples and characterization of their components [13]. Fluorescence spectroscopy can also be applied in determining the bitterness of beer and the presence of vitamin B_2 and other aromatic compounds along with the storage study [14]. Chemometric methods are applied for analyzing the data obtained for quantitative as well as qualitative information of sample product properties. Excitation–emission matrix (EEM) in fluorescence spectroscopy is combined with various chemometric techniques, which works in multiway for classification as well as the characterization of beer and its components. Difference is found in the fingerprints of undiluted and diluted beer samples. Parallel factor analysis (PARAFAC) and k-nearest neighbor (k-NN) as well as other discriminant analysis techniques are also utilized [15]. This chapter deals with the fundamental concept and characteristics of fluorescence and types of fluorescence spectra, factors affecting fluorescence spectra, and their application for characterizing the quality of beer samples.

3.2 Concept of fluorescence

Fluorescence is a nonthermal process that takes place by emission of light by living or nonliving objects after absorption of light. The light generated is cold as compared to the hot light. Some of the molecules go further to an electronically excited state after absorbing Vis or UV light and return to the ground state by emitting photons that have distinct energy than that of absorbed radiation. The molecules can return to the ground state in three different ways, namely, photoluminescence, fluorescence, and phosphorescence. The phenomenon of fluorescence is demonstrated via Jablonski's energy diagram (Fig. 3.1). Many of the molecules that are at room temperature attain very low vibrational energy of

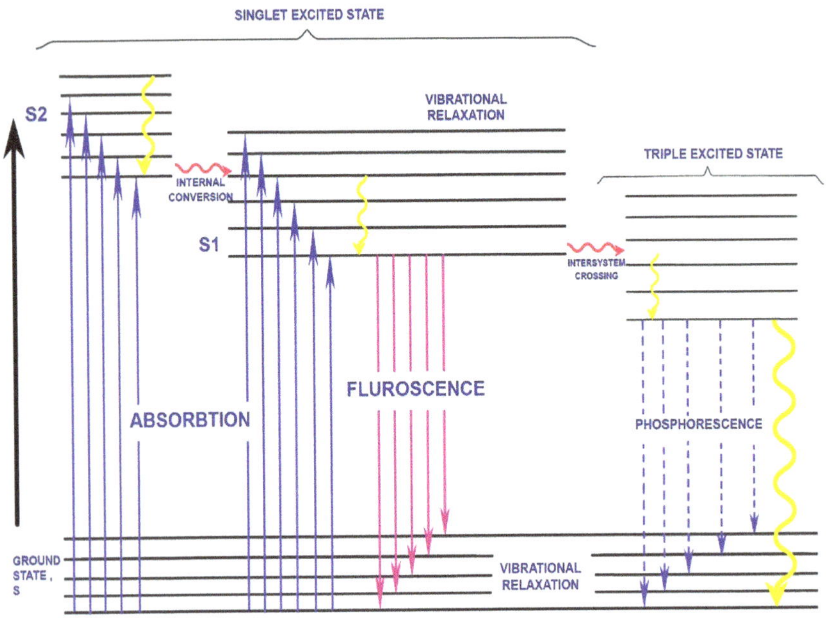

Figure 3.1 Jablonski's energy diagram.

fundamental electronic ground state (S_0) [16]. A molecule absorbs a photon and gets excited and reaches to vibrationally higher states of energy levels. New molecules are in excited state viz. singlet states shown by S_x, where x = 1, 2, etc. Every molecule gets excited for a significant time period, and this process is very fast (10^{-15} s). In the next step, either internal conversion or vibration relaxation takes place, which deactivates the molecules that were in the excited state to the ground state of the singlet state (S_1). Many different processes are competing, which results in the deactivation of molecules from S_1 to the S_0 ground state. The transition of molecules from S_1 to S_0 (10^{-11}–10^{-9} s) is usually the non-radiative transition and crossing of the intersystem to the triplet state (10^{-10}–10^{-8} s). Finally, the fluorescence emission takes place in the range of emission of photon, which is called fluorescence (10^{-10}–10^{-7} s) [17]. The wavelength of emission is more than the wavelength of excitation due to the loss of energy, which is known as the Stokes shift. Fluorescent molecules are denoted as the fluorophores, made of aromatic closed-chain molecules linked with π-bond electronic configuration.

3.3 Characteristics of fluorescence

The photons get emitted, showing transition from S_1 to S_0, or numerous transitions between states is characterized as fluorescence. Mostly, the fluorescence occurs from the S_1 state, and thus, its attributes are not dependent on the excitation wavelength. The Stokes rule states that the spectrum of fluorescence is switched to the higher wavelength having lower energy with regard to the spectrum of absorption as part of the energy absorbed is vanished during the relaxation of the excited state. The Stokes shift ($\Delta\overline{\nu}$) wavelength is defined as:

$$\Delta\overline{\nu} = \overline{\nu}_{abs} - \overline{\nu}_{em} \tag{3.1}$$

Where $\overline{\nu}_{abs}$ is the maximum-wavelength band of the absorption spectra, and $\overline{\nu}_{em}$ is the maximum-wavelength band of the fluorescence spectra. The reciprocal of Stokes shift wavelength is called Stokes shift wavenumber, and these are the characteristic of a specific molecule [17]. The fluorescent compounds are characterized by two main attributes, namely, quantum yield and the lifetime. The fluorescence quantum yield is defined as the ratio of the number of photons that are emitted over the entire spectrum of fluorescence to the number of photons that are absorbed. The fluorescence lifetime is the average time that the molecule spends in the excited state. Fluorescence shows anisotropic behavior, which can also be stated as the measure of the rate and the degree of rotational repositioning of a molecule, during the time interval between both the transitions (absorption and emission). The attributes of fluorescence depend on the properties and structure of the molecule and its environment.

3.4 Factors affecting fluorescence phenomenon

Fluorescence is exhibited by only few compounds. Organic compounds that possess fluorescent character have alternate C = C double bonds with firm molecular skeleton and aromatic character. Fluorescent compounds comprise heterocyclic compounds, polyaromatic hydrocarbons, and some highly unsaturated aliphatic compounds. The compounds having characteristics of fluorescence are influenced by the position as well as nature of constituents in a molecule. Fluorescence is very responsive to the environment of the molecule that is in emittance mode, and the magnitude of this responsiveness depends upon fluorophores [16]. The impact of the microenvironment results in changes in the magnitude of the intensity of fluorescence and further leads to the shifting of fluorescence maxima (blue or red). In some of the cases, changes in intensity are followed by shifting in the fluorescence spectrum as well. Fluorophores at polar points are highly sensitive to the local environment polarity. The shift in the pH affects the dissociation very strongly or disturbs the protonation equilibria and alters the rate at which nonradiative processes compete with the fluorescence molecule, further affecting the lifetimes and quantum yields. Temperature has an impact on the dynamic quenching, which in turn affects the signals of fluorescence [18].

As the fluorescence quenching declines, the excited molecules get deactivated, which results in the decrease in the fluorescence intensity. Quenching may comprise either inter- or intramolecular interactions, including energy dissipation, excited-state reactions, collisional deactivation, molecular rearrangements, etc. [9]. Energy transfer in the form of resonance represents the quenching process that leads to interaction directly between the acceptor and donor molecule, which leads to either partial or full inactivation of the excited donor fluorophore with no emission of light [18].

Similarly, in the ground-state complex formation, the fluorescence intensity of a sample was decreased due to repression of the fluorophores in the ground state. However, in this process, no quenching takes place, as there is no formation of excited state of the fluorophore. This makes the process of quenching mechanically dissimilar to the excited-state quenching. Fluorescence can be developed intermolecularly as well by impeding an intramolecular technique of quenching or modifying the ground states of fluorophores. Some of the factors such as the presence of quenchers and properties of the local microenvironment have a great impact on the measured signals of fluorescence. Thus, the utilization of apt methods for determining and analyzing the fluorescence data gives important information, about fluorescent compounds and sample matrix. The responsiveness of the fluorophores to the current circumstances has been studied extensively, making a base for scrutinizing the characteristics of fluorescence in a microenvironment [17]. In ratiometric fluorescence, the intensities are determined at two or more wavelengths in the emission or excitation spectrum to find some modifications in the local environment. The fluorescence probes have been used to measure pressure, temperature, metal ion concentration, viscosity, and polarity, along with nitrogen/oxygen reactive enzymes and species [19]. Intensity of fluorescence in the diluted solutions is determined by the following expression:

$$I_F(\lambda_{em}, \lambda_{exc}) = 2.3 \quad kI_0(\lambda_{exc})\Phi_\lambda(\lambda_{em})\varepsilon(\lambda_{exc})cl \tag{3.2}$$

Here, I_F = intensity of fluorescence, Φ_λ = quantum yield of fluorescence, I_0 = intensity of incident light, ε = coefficient of molar absorption, k = proportionality factor, c = molar concentration of the fluorophore, I = sample length of optical path, λ_{em} = emission wavelength, λ_{exc} = excitation wavelength.

Intensity of fluorescence depends upon fluorophore concentration, quantum yield, and molar absorptivity. The intensity of fluorescence is directly proportional to the concentration of fluorophore in lower optical density solutions (absorbance <0.05), but linear proportionality is affected by the inner filter effects. These rely on the conditions of measurement, which reduces the intensity of fluorescence for higher concentrations of fluorophores. When there is exorbitant absorption of incident light followed by reabsorption of emitted light, the intensity of fluorescence decreases in concentrated solutions.

Eq. (3.2) includes the base for the traditional implementation of fluorometric methods. Concentration of unknown samples was determined by using calibration curve drawn between the intensity of fluorescence versus concentration of the standard solutions of a specific analyte. However, this traditional strategy may be used only for evaluation of simple samples, especially monofluorophoric. If the sample is complex, then sample pretreatment is required. In case of techniques of absorption, two beams of light are taken, and their intensities are collated, whereas in fluorescence, the measurement of light intensity is carried out against a dark background. Therefore, fluorometry is a highly sensitive technique as compared to the absorption spectrometry, which measures even the femtomolar concentration of the analytes [19].

3.5 Fluorescence spectra and its types

Fluorescence spectroscopy measures the spectral distribution of intensity of emitted light. In the model system of a single fluorophore, the fluorescence is totally characterized by traditional excitation and emission spectra of a specific compound. The characterization of complex and real samples (multifluorophoric) has been reported to require more futuristic techniques for measurement [19]. The two main types of spectra achieved using spectrofluorometer are excitation and emission spectra of fluorescence, which are adequate for characterizing single fluorophore model systems. While viewing the emission spectrum, the wavelength of the excitation radiation is not changed, and then, the spectral distribution of the radiation emitted is recoded as a function of the wavelength of emission. Furthermore, viewing an excitation spectrum, the signal of fluorescence is recorded at a particular wavelength of the emission monochromator by scanning the excitation wavelength, and a compound can show fluorescence if it absorbs a photon. Thus, the excitation spectrum ascertains the wavelength of light that is absorbed by the compound. As a result, spectrum of a molecule in excitation mode must be similar to its absorption spectrum of UV−Vis radiation, having same positions of maxima along with shape. The shape and position of the excitation as well as emission spectra in a monofluorophoric system are not dependent on emission and excitation wavelength, respectively. The variations in the emission or excitation spectra with studied wavelength in such system indicate the presence of impurities, emission from a variety dissimilar to the absorbing one or the involvement of excited-state reactions. Different kinds of fluorescence spectra are excitation spectra, emission spectra, 3D spectra involving EEM, synchronous fluorescence spectra, and front-face spectra [16].

3.5.1 Total luminescence spectra

Undiluted samples of beer showed high absorption of UV−Vis radiation, and thus, the fluorescence that is measured by applying the right-angled geometry is seriously disturbed because of primary as well as secondary inner filter effects. Front-face geometry must avoid the effects of filter, although other events including transfer of energy and collisional quenching are not removed. Appropriate dilution of the sample must be done as it minimizes intensities of fluorescence energy from those compounds. These samples are present in lower concentrations, or they have small quantum yields of fluorescence.

3.5.2 Excitation spectra

An excitation spectrum indicates a disparity in the emission spectra, which is analyzed at decided wavelength, whereas the wavelength of excitation progresses over a smaller or longer range of wavelength. Best installation of the instrument must give the light to be excited as near as possible to the spectrum of absorption of the fluorophore. From time to time, the corrections should be done, as the spectrum of excitation is disrupted by variation in the intensity of incident light with the wavelength. Thus, the improved excitation spectrum is similar to the spectrum of absorption when the solution that is being analyzed has single molecular species present in the ground state. As there are many molecular species or many states of chemical oxidation or single species having a state of protonation–deprotonation, both excitation and absorption spectra, which are corrected, cannot superimpose each other (Fig. 3.2).

3.5.3 Emission spectra

Spectrum showing emission has the possibility of distribution of many transitions from least vibration level of S_1 toward various vibration level of S_0. Therefore it is commensurate to a divergence of the intensity of luminescence light emission, which is presented as a function of the excitation wavelength (Fig. 3.2). A fluorescence spectrum of emission is distinctive of a particular compound given.

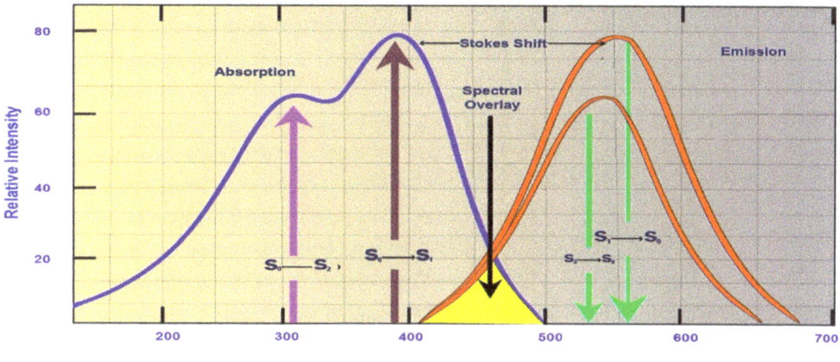

Figure 3.2 Schematic diagram of excitation emission spectra.

3.5.4 3D fluorescence spectra

3D fluorescence spectroscopy is also called as EEM spectroscopy. When the monochromators are arranged sequentially possessing excitation and emission spectra, it is feasible to analyze emission spectra for distinct wavelengths of excitation. As a result, the assemblage of emission spectra occurs at distinct wavelengths of excitation. Thus, the EEM attained has two major dimensions: emission and excitation wavelengths. Matrices of fluorescence give a variety of fluorescence maps of fluorophores, which are present in a mixture allowing associated characterization of them.

3.5.5 Synchronous fluorescence spectra

Synchronous fluorescence spectra (SFS) are advantageous as they are capable of characterizing various fluorophores from one spectrum, which strikes a balance between EEM spectra and standard accession of emission as well as excitation fluorescence spectra. SFS is different from EEM spectra, as a wavelength difference, which is fixed ($\Delta\lambda$) between the emission (λ_{em}) and excitation wavelength (λ_{ex}), is used for spectral accession, and the restraint ($\lambda_{em} = \Delta\lambda + \lambda_{ex}$) is also kept in mind [20]. The spectrum is found out at the excitation wavelengths (λ_{ex1}, λ_{ex2}, ..., λ_{exj}), and emission wavelengths can be calculated as: $\lambda_{em1} = \lambda_{ex1} + \Delta\lambda$; $\lambda_{em2} = \lambda_{ex2} + \Delta\lambda$, etc. Synchronous spectra are seen as a slanted band of the emission–excitation surface (Fig. 3.3). $\Delta\lambda$, also called as offset, can be changed whenever required [21]. In accordance with the mode of

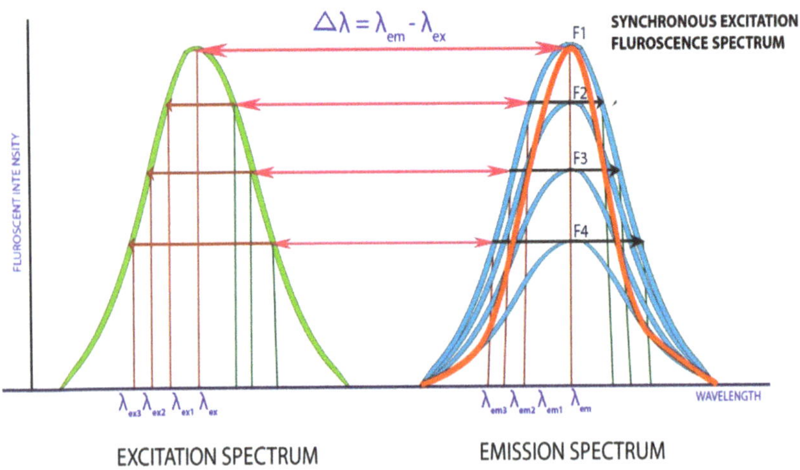

Figure 3.3 Schematic diagram of synchronous fluorescence spectra.

scanning, between the monochromators of excitation and emission, three main spectral varieties of synchronous fluorescence are detected [22]. Scanning of the emission and excitation monochromator is attained by using a wavelength shift $\Delta\lambda$, which must be constant, along with a shift in constant energy ($\Delta\nu$) or frequency or at various speeds. If there is variation in the "offset" with the same pitch, a partial 3D spectrum is achieved [23]. SFS is advantageous as it furnishes complete information on the fluorophore mixture, which facilitates the production of finer spectral bands; it reduces the changes in spectra for a given analyte. This simplifies the emission spectra, and it also compensates for Rayleigh and Raman scattering. SFS is generally used for characterization of several mixtures, and it has immense applications in food industries [24]. The instrument is organized optically, and the sample is analyzed that needs inclination in accordance with the exciting light.

3.5.5.1 Right-angled fluorescence

When light moves across the sample, disruption in the fluorescence can be seen by the absorbance phenomena (Fig. 3.4A). Thus, the sample should be diluted so as to get the absorbance below 0.05. This type of fluorescence is not appropriate for opaque solids, samples with high viscosity, and powders.

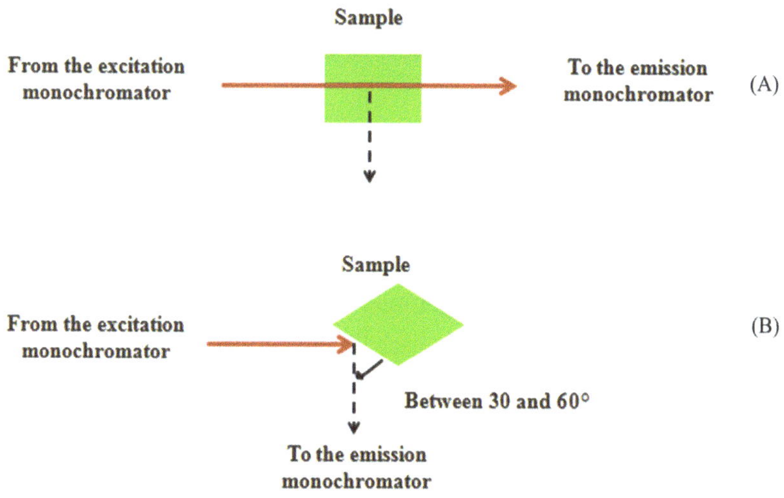

Figure 3.4 (A) Right-angled fluorescence (B) Front-face fluorescence.

3.5.5.2 *Front-face fluorescence*

In order to evade absorption and dilution problems, the solution having the sample is presented under the incident light at an acute angle, so as to perform the measurements in a similar manner as done in attenuated total reflectance—infrared spectroscopy. There is a special mode of recording in the infrared spectroscopy, which applies a crystal as a support for short-lived wave transmission generated by exciting light above the sample holder of crystal from the viewpoint of incidence angle (Fig. 3.4B). Emission and excitation take place optically on the surface of the cuvette that is alike where light enters by a few microns. The sample can be nontransparent, but it should be analogous, because the characteristics of the surface will represent the complete sample [25].

3.6 Phenomena of fluorescence scattering

The scattering observes two interactions of light and matter known as Raman and Rayleigh scattering. Data obtained by fluorescence are usually afflicted by both of these scattering processes, which can cause disturbance in modeling of data of fluorescence by PARAFAC model. These scattering signals cause problem in the decomposition of signals of fluorescence, and their effect must be reduced [26]. It is important to know about these scattering signals for further analysis of beer samples.

3.6.1 Raman scattering

It is also known as the linkage between photons appearing from a source of light that is monochromatic and molecules within the sample. Many photons at $1/10^8$ will be dispersed inelastically, suffering from the loss of energy corresponding to the vibrational transition. This type of scattering takes place when the electric field present in the excited form causes a change in the polarization of the molecule. It can determine the changes in polarization effectively during the vibration of heteronuclear or homoskeletons. It results in an emission that is weak, and it can interfere or it can get perplexed with the sample fluorescence, which is usually much weaker than the Rayleigh scattering (Fig. 3.5). Signal of fluorescence is not covered by Raman scattering, but its orientation can lead to distortion of signal [27]. The use of Raman interaction as the main signal of the

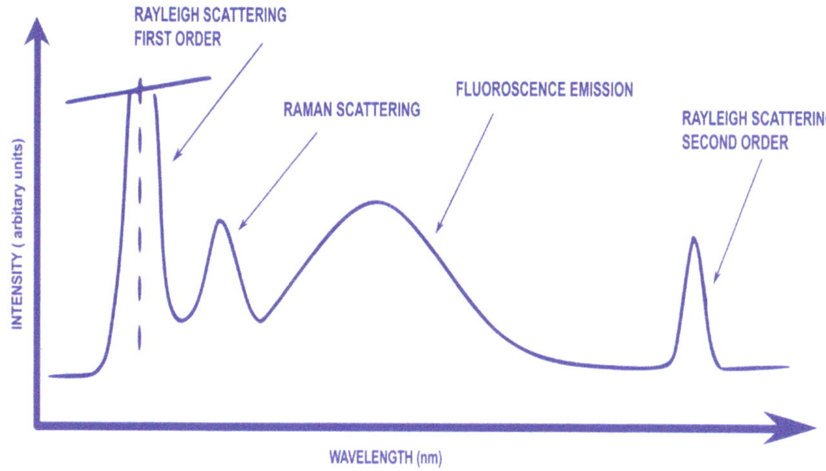

Figure 3.5 Schematic diagram of fluorescence and scattering.

molecule has developed Raman spectroscopy, which adjuncts infrared spectroscopy. There may be variation in chemical bond polarization of like the dipole moment, which incites the bonds, and there may be formation of persistent dipole moment of chemical bonds. Interaction of light and matter causes specific vibrations to get activated in either Raman or infrared spectroscopy or both. Raman spectroscopy can be applied for the determination of structures of chemicals, conformation of molecular arrangements, molecular configuration, and the analysis of molecular orientation or inter- and intramolecular forces.

3.6.2 Rayleigh scattering

It is the scattering process of the interacting wave and matter because of an elastic collision taking place between electrons and photons in the molecule. The photons are scattered with the help of electrons, which are way smaller than the wavelength of incidence. Electrons bounding to an atom or molecule scatter photons, and the incident wave forms electric field that distorts the cloud of atoms of the electron, and the negative charges possesses center of gravity that fluctuates with respect to the nucleus having positive charge. Due to this phenomenon, a dipole is formed, which causes induced radiation known as Rayleigh scattering. The law of Rayleigh states that intensity that is dispersed by a medium is inversely proportional to the fourth power of the wavelength of the incident light ($1/\lambda^4$), which implies that when the wavelength is lower, the radiation is more and will be scattered more as well as the scattered light intensity will be very high. Wavelengths that are found in the ultraviolet range get dispersed more, and thus, it is less transmitted than those in the spectrum of infrared rays. Photons get dispersed when the wavelengths of excitation and emission are the same, and there is no loss of energy. Rayleigh scattering does not carry any chemical information about the medium being analyzed, and it can disrupt the fluorescence phenomenon of compounds of interest by restricting the responsivity, especially for wavelengths near to the excitation wavelength. It can be contemplated as a remnant, which must be eliminated so as to gain access of the fluorescence signals of the molecules that are targeted.

3.7 Fluorescence geometry of beer

The attributes of beer fluorescence are supposed to be extremely complicated due to overlapping of emissions from various species. Thus, it is important to study techniques of multidimensional fluorescence to get a thorough knowledge of the fluorescent component. 3D spectra are also called as EEM or luminescence of total spectra, where one axis shows the excitation wavelength and another shows wavelength of emission, and the third wavelength shows the intensity. On the other hand, 3D spectra may be altered into 2D contour maps, where one axis shows the emission and another shows the excitation wavelength. Plotting of the contours is done by attaching the points of fluorescence intensity that are equal, and it is practically more important for visual examination of the fluorescence patterns. TLS gives a complete illustration of the fluorescent elements present in the mixture, integrating all the details present in the fluorescence and absorption spectra of fluorescent elements. Because of these attributes, the TLS counter map serves as a fingerprint that is unique for character classification and sample identification. The spectral alignment of the EEM depends on the number of common emissions in the excitation wavelengths used to form the contour plots. Thus, many emission scans for each sample are needed for accession of contour plots of adequate resolution on the common spectrofluorometers. The evaluation may be paced up with the charged couple device of video spectrofluorometers [28]. Instead of TLS, SFS would be more useful for analyzing fluorescent elements. Both the emission and excitation attributes are involved in the spectrum and concurrently scanning both the spectrums and maintaining a regular distance between them. Samples of undiluted beer show high UV–Vis absorption, and the fluorescence is analyzed by applying the common method; the right-angled geometry is critically disturbed because of primary as well as secondary inner filter effects, which can be removed by dilution. Dilution also reduces the intensities of fluorescence emerging from the compounds that are either present or less in concentration or have low quantum yield of fluorescence. Undiluted samples can be analyzed by applying the back- or front-face geometry [29]. This geometry evades filter effects, while other phenomena like collisional quenching and energy transfer remains active. The triangular cell of this geometry reduces the path of radiation, which results in decrease of primary inner filter effect. Even at this shorter path length, the emitted light is still absorbed with maximum absorption of shorter excitation wavelength. Therefore, all the three geometries were used in fluorescence analysis of beer: right angle for samples that are diluted, and front and back face for bulk samples [13]. Front-face geometry showed almost complete fluorescent characteristics of beer (undiluted) and its spectra showed an intense band with the excitation and emission at wavelengths of 250 and 350 nm, respectively. In addition to intense band, a distinct emission band and less-intense emission band with emission and excitation and n was also observed at 350 and 420 nm and 450 and 520 nm, respectively. The diluted beer spectra showed short-wavelength excitation at 250 nm and emission at 350 nm. The additional spectra of weak-emission band excitation at 350 nm and emission at 420 nm were also observed. Usually, no fluorescence is observed above the excitation of 400 nm and emission of 500 nm [13]. The analysis of undiluted beer using back-face geometry method showed disappearance of short-wavelength emission; however, longer-wavelength emission was present in reasonable intensity. Several lager beer samples were analyzed and showed the presence of quite similar fluorescent elements in the emission spectra [13]. The intensity as well as shape of synchronous spectra depend upon the offset between the emission and excitation wavelengths, $\Delta\lambda$, which is the wavelength interval of the emission and absorption spectra. Synchronous fluorescence spectra of an undiluted beer in front-face geometry at $\Delta\lambda = 10$ nm showed a sharp band with a maximum at 283 nm and a weak emission at 385, 426, and 488 nm [13]. The short-wavelength band of emission is expanded in the spectra at $\Delta\lambda = 30$ nm and maxima obtained at 275 nm, and broad emission was observed between 300 and 500 nm. Furthermore, the intensity of fluorescence in the region of short-wavelength decreases, and if the wavelength is increased by 60–80 nm and the intensity of long wavelength band grows, their maxima is then shifted to the blue. The SFS of undiluted beer samples in back-face geometry were absent with the short-wavelength emission.

3.8 Beer constituents having fluorescent properties

Major components of beer, ethanol, carbohydrates, and water are nonfluorescent, but beer contains a broad spectrum of minor components that includes proteins, vitamins, amino acids, carbohydrates, and phenolic compounds that show fluorescence. The inherent emission of beers initiates from various fluorescent species. The complete task of the spectral attributes is complicated. Some provisional assignments of quality can be done, which is based on the difference of the features discerned with the well-known properties of fluorescence, the specific beer constituents. The fluorescence properties and detected concentration of some of the beer constituents are shown in Table 3.1, which may fluctuate broadly,

Table 3.1 Concentration, excitation, and emission wavelengths of fluorophores present in beer.

Types of fluorophores	Excitation wavelength (nm)	Emission wavelength (nm)	Concentration of fluorophores
Vitamins			
Riboflavin (Vit. B_2)	270, 382, 448	518 [18]	0.021–0.043 mg/100 g [36] 0.0158–0.0279 mg/100 g [37] 0.216–0.313 mg/dm^3 [10]
FAD	262, 370, 450	540 [38]	0.021–0.068 mg/dm^3 [39] 0.0013–0.0054 mg/100 g [37]
FMN	265, 370, 450	540 [38]	0.086 mg/dm^3 [39]
NAD(P)H (Vit.B_3)	340	470 [30]	0.69–1.4 mg/100 g [36]

(*Continued*)

Table 3.1 (Continued)

Types of fluorophores	Excitation wavelength (nm)	Emission wavelength (nm)	Concentration of fluorophores
Pyridoxine (Vit.B_6)	328	393 [18]	0.05–0.09 mg/100 g [36]
Amino acids			
Tryptophan	280	357 [18]	3.3 mg/100 g [36]
Phenylalanine	258	284 [18]	6.1 mg/100 g [36] 20.3–105.7 mg/dm^3 [40]
Tyrosine	276	302 [18]	15.2 mg/100 g [36] 5.8–71.5 mg/dm^3 [40]
Phenolic compounds			
Ferulic acid	340	460 [41]	6.9 mg/dm^3 [41] 13.54 mg/dm^3 [42]
Epicatechin	280	320–324 [43]	65.7 mg/dm^3 [41] 0.9–2.2 mg/dm^3 [32]
Catechin	280	320–324 [43]	3.5–6.5 mg/dm^3 [32]
p- Coumaric acid	330	435 [44]	2.3 mg/dm^3 [41] 1.08 mg/dm^3 [42]
Gallic acid	260	357 [41]	3.1 mg/dm^3 [41]

depending on the type of beer. The compounds showing natural fluorescence belong to three different groups of components of beer: vitamins, phenolic compounds, and amino acids. An intense band is found in each beer sample with emission at c. 300–400 nm and excitation at c. 250–300 nm, which has been accredited to amino acids [11]. A variety of amino acids are found in beer, and among them, only three (phenylalanine, tryptophan, and tyrosine) are fluorescent and have aromatic character. Short-wavelength region emission can be originated from epicatechin (proanthocyanidin) or catechin. Participation of polyphenols at this zone of spectrum is very less, and their removal by polyvinyl polypyrrolidone does not affect the detected fluorescence significantly [10]. The wide emission at longer wavelength emerges from various fluorescent compounds including phenolic compounds and vitamin B group [11]. Beer possesses several phenolic compounds that comprise a vast horizon of structures from monophenols that are simple to polyphenols (polymeric) having different problems, and beer is also an affluent source of vitamin B (water soluble). Vitamin B_2 emission is observed at the band of emission at c. 450–500/600 nm [30]. Mainly flavin adenine dinucleotides (FAD), riboflavin, flavin mononucleotide (FMN) are naturally found in vitamin B, but beer mainly contains riboflavin. Vitamin B_3 (niacin) involves nicotinamide, nicotinic acid along with their coenzyme (nicotinamide adenine dinucleotide phosphate (NADP) and nicotinamide adenine dinucleotide (NAD)). Some of the fluorescent compounds include minimized forms of NAD(P)H and vitamin B_6 group comprises pyridoxal, pyridoxine, pyridoxic acid, pyridoxamine, pyridoxal-5-phosphate, and all the compounds show emission in the range of 385–400 nm. According to Apperson et al. [10], iso-α- acids also contribute to autofluorescence of beer. The profound emission bands of short wavelength are seen in the spectra of synchronous fluorescence of diluted samples of beer, ascribed to amino acid fluorescence, especially tyrosine, which is similar to spectra of total luminescence. The emission of long wavelength in the synchronous spectra of beer must arise from compounds of vitamin B group. Presence of numerous bands tells that various substances, especially phenolic compounds, emit in this region, whereas tryptophan, phenylalanine, and tyrosine show a single band in the short-wavelength region with their maxima at 296, 263, and 283 nm, respectively. Emission of riboflavin takes place in the long-wavelength region with the maximum spectra at 489 nm. Amino acid concentration in beer can be an indicator for the performance of fermentation. Wort contains free amino acids, which get metabolized by yeast during the process of fermentation, and hence, the amount of amino acids in beer is found by wort metabolism [31]. Phenolic compounds are either harmful or beneficial to various beer properties [32]. They help in chemical as well as physical stability, foam maintenance, and shelf life, and they also provide flavor by giving astringency and bitterness to beer. Polyphenols help in polyphenol–protein haze development. Many phenolic compounds act as antioxidants also in our body, which contributes toward good health. Vitamins enhance the nutritional value of beer, and its active forms serve as the prosthetic groups of oxidoreductase enzymes that causes important reduction/oxidation steps in near about all the metabolic pathways [33]. Riboflavin possesses many disease-preventing and health-promoting functions, which help in prevention from malaria, certain cancers, and vascular diseases. It protects important tissues from oxidative injury, which results from stroke or heart attack [34]. It contributes nutritionally along with the enhancement of flavor changes: stale flavor and sunstruck [35].

3.9 Application of fluorescence spectroscopy in beer

Fluorescence spectroscopy is widely used for the quantification of functional chemical compounds and bioactive compounds of various beverages such as juice, wine, beer, and brandy. Various compounds in beer such as riboflavin, polyphenols, caramel, caffeine, and aromatic amino acids were analyzed using fluorescence spectroscopy. As these compounds affect the nutritional and organoleptic quality of beer, therefore fluorescence spectroscopy also helps in differentiating various types of beer [45].

3.9.1 Stratification of beer

SFS of individual beers shows variation by generating unique spectral patterns and can be used to study qualitative parameters for monitoring of quality for describing or authenticating beer types [13]. Multivariate statistical methods must be practiced, and exploratory analysis of SFS of several beers is performed through principle component analysis (PCA) [46]. SFS method can be used for describing different beers based on the spectra by applying two statistical methods like linear discriminant analysis (LDA) or the k-NN method [13]. LDA is performed on the simple datasets, and for this objective near about six wavelengths are taken from spectrum of synchronous fluorescence, which is determined at a specific wavelength ($\Delta\lambda$) and analyzed. LDA also shows satisfactory discrimination between different beers. There is no need to observe the entire spectra for discrimination, but only selected fluorescence intensity is seen at selected EEM.

The k-NN method is a type of nonparametric method that helps in the analysis of the whole spectra without reducing any of the datasets [47]. In this process, mainly the test object is designated to a group, which is mostly depicted in the set of k-nearest training objects. Among all the data points, the nearest data points are called the nearest neighbors, and further, the judgment is done according to the values attained by these neighbors. k-NN method is the simplest machine learning technique as all the work is done by the classifier by observing examples that are almost akin to the one that has to be classified, and values of k are selected in the range of 1–10. Arrangement of several beer samples by using k-NN method is outstanding with very low or zero classification error with very less values of standard deviation [13]. The best insight can be gained for bulk beers using SFS, measuring at $\Delta\lambda = 10$ and 60 nm along with diluted beers at $\Delta\lambda = 10$ nm. Short as well as long wavelengths of UV and Vis emission, respectively, are capable of discriminating various beer samples. Both of these techniques can be used for analyzing beer samples, but the spectra of bulky samples are more authentic than diluted beers. Along with qualitative differences, samples have different fluorescence intensities of specific components. All these dissimilarities must show fluorescent components and must be utilized for quantitative assessment of beer components.

3.9.2 Bitterness of beer

The presence of iso-α- acids is because of the hop, and it is the regular analysis in the industry of brewery. As bitterness is an essential parameter of quality. Christenin et al. [11] suggested two methods of fluorescence for determination of bitterness in beer quantitatively. First method studied the EEM of beer via autofluorescence. This process needs dilution and then degassing only prior to measurements. Regression model for partial least square (PLS) multivariate analysis was carried out, and the bitterness of the sample in terms of international bitterness unit (IBU) was measured using six components of PLS model [48]. Another process for determining the bitterness of beer was the delayed fluorescence with europium by incorporating ions of lanthanide to the samples of beer [11]. Chelation of some of the lanthanide ions and iso-α- acids having carbonyl structure along with few unique fluorescent properties of the complex, etc., causes delayed fluorescence.

3.9.3 Vitamin B analysis of beer

Determination of Vitamin B in beer samples is very important for nutritional aspect and stability of flavor. Native fluorophores of vitamin B are used for determining its quantity in beer samples. Generally, riboflavin is found in large quantities in beer as compared to other vitamin B like flavin. Enzymatic or microbiological methods were used for vitamin B determination, and later, it was substituted by High Performance Liquid Chromatography (HPLC) method. Currently, the determination of fluorophores at excitation and emission wavelengths helps in evaluating vitamin B content in beer sample [49]. A PLS regression model was developed, and calibration was done using SF spectra and emission spectra of riboflavin content found by fluorometric titration. These regression models showed better ability to determine the concentration of riboflavin present in beer samples. PLS-1 and

PLS-2 methods were used to draw calibration models, which were made by data obtained from SF and EEM spectra of beer [48].

3.9.4 Storage analysis of beer

Fluorescence spectroscopy can also help investigate changes in the composition of beer during storage. Fresh bear showing total luminescence spectra along with stored beer (in light) differs mostly in the band observed at 450 nm in the excitation and in between 500–600 nm in the emission spectrum. This is the zone determined for vitamin B_2 (riboflavin) and is ascribed to flavins found in beer, but when exposed to light, this type of emission disappears due to photodegradation of flavins [50]. The change occurring while storage is more prominent in the bulk samples of beer than in the diluted ones. When there is a need to monitor the quality of beer samples, then the product is separated into classes like aged and fresh samples. The k-NN and LDA methods are used based on their fluorescence spectra. The classification error increases at greater values of k and rate of misclassification is higher for spectra measured for $\Delta\lambda = 60$ nm, and LDA method gives 100% categorization for both the sets of synchronous spectra. Changes in the intrinsic beer fluorescence occur during the aging process, which refers to minor and subtle chemical changes of components of beer. A thorough knowledge of mixture of fluorescent compounds is gained, and then studies are further required to define all the specific molecules. It is possible that validated and stored fluorescence spectra may serve as a reference for the purpose of quality control of beer. Investigation of the processes occurring in beer samples can be seen when the sample is exposed to light. When the beer sample is exposed to the visible light, it might give a flavor known as "lightstruck," because of the emergence of 3-methyl-2-butene-1-thiol (MBT) [35]. The formation of this flavor takes place due to the excitation of riboflavin to its triplet state, and electron transport also takes place from iso-α-acids [51]. Estimation of light-induced breakdown of beer components mainly focuses on the development of sulfur-containing compounds, degrading in nature and used particularly in formation of MBT. Quantitative analysis of MBT shows a great challenge because its threshold for flavor is very low, it has a relatively high boiling point (126°C), chemical reactivity, and aptness to adsorb onto the surface. Fluorescence enables the analysis of tryptophan along with catechin, providing some protection against light-struck flavor formation [52].

3.10 Quality analysis of beer using PARAFAC model

A multidimensional chemometric technique like PARAFAC has been being used for chemometric analysis of spectra of beer fluorescence. Kahle et al. [53] used PARAFAC model and studied fluorescence of eight samples of beer by explaining three components. PARAFAC is most widely used algorithm to carry out the EEM calculations, and fluorescence EEM measurements should provide an output in the form of a data matrix. During the measurement of several samples, each of the matrixes is added to a three-way array. If the sample is calculated at K excitation wavelengths and J emission wavelengths, then the fluorescent intensities obtained should be collected in a matrix of size J x K. I denotes the number of samples that are measured, then the three-way array is build up (I x J x K) for measuring samples (I). This array is further used for the PARAFAC modeling in multiway. The direction of sample in correspondence to the matrix rows is known as the first mode; emission mode is the second mode, and excitation mode is the third mode. PARAFAC modeling breaks an array of three-way into a set of trilinear terms by reducing the sum of squares of the residuals (e_{ijk}), which shows variations that are unexplained [54].

$$x_{ijk} = \sum_{r=0}^{R} a_{ir} b_{jr} c_{kr} + e_{ijk}$$

where, $i = 1, \ldots, I$; $j = 1, \ldots, J$; $k = 1, \ldots, K$; $r = 1, \ldots, R$. The PARAFAC model is explained by loading matrices A, B, and C having elements a_{ir}, b_{jr}, and c_{kr}, respectively. In the above equation, x_{ijk} commensurate to one data point in three-way array for ith sample, along with jth and kth variables on modes 2 and 3, respectively. "R" corresponds to the number of components of PARAFAC model. All the components in the model are denoted by values of a, b, and c. The PARAFAC model shows fluorescence present in the complex system, and it has all the information about related concentration of fluorophore in each sample. The parameters show pure spectra of emission as well as excitation of fluorophores that are modeled. Evaluation of a number of constituents in the PARAFAC model of the EEM's of beers and the affirmation that proper assessment is done by the validation of model through the split- half analysis and core consistency diagnostics [55].

3.11 Conclusions

Fluorescence is a nonthermal process that takes place by emission of light by living or nonliving objects after absorption of light. Fluorescence spectroscopy is used for the determination of oxidation in fish, meat, and for other assay of milk, cheeses, and edible oils. The fluorescent analysis is beneficial due to the existence of natural fluorescent components of food or its contaminants. Various fluorescing components of beer can be used for analyzing beer components using EEM spectra. This technology can be extensively used for characterization of beer, and it can also help determine the changes in the beer components during storage, which can enhance the keeping quality of beer. PARAFAC modeling technique is extensively used for measuring sensitive components in the beer with more accurate results in a short period of time. Spectroscopic method has also been used to monitor changes in production as well as during storage of beer, providing noninvasive calculations. Further, more fluorescent compounds must be identified to know about in-depth knowledge of components responsible for quality characteristics of beer.

References

[1] G.A. DaSilva, F. Augusto, R.J. Poppi, Exploratory analysis of the volatile profile of beers by HS-SPME-GC, Food Chem. 111 (2008) 1057–1063.
[2] H.E. Anderson, I.C. Santos, Z.L. Hildenbrand, K.A. Schug, A review of the analytical methods used for beer ingredient and finished product analysis and quality control, Anal. Chim. Acta 1085 (2019) 1–20. Available from: https://doi.org/10.1016/j.aca.2019.07.061.
[3] S. Cortacero-Ramirez, M.H.B. de Castro, A. Segura-Carretero, C. Cruces-Blanco, A. Fernandez-Gutierrez, Analysis of beer components by capillary electrophoretic methods, Trends Anal. Chem. 22 (2003) 440–455.
[4] V.R. Preedy, Beer in Health and Disease Prevention, Academic Press, 2008. ISBN: 978-0-12-373891-2.
[5] P.B. Oldham, M.E. Mc Carroll, L.B. Mc Gown, I.M. Warner, Molecular fluorescence, phosphorescence, and chemiluminescence spectrometry, Anal. Chem. 72 (2000) 197R–209R.
[6] T. Ndou, I. Warner, Applications of multidimensional absorption and luminescence spectroscopies in analytical chemistry, Chem. Rev. 91 (4) (1991) 493–507. Available from: https://doi.org/10.1021/cr00004a003.
[7] E. Sikorska, K. Wojcicki, W. Kozak, A. Gliszczynska-Swiglo, I. Khmelinskii, T. Gorecki, et al., Front-Face fluorescence spectroscopy and chemometrics for quality control of cold-pressed rapeseed oil during storage, Foods 8 (665) (2019) 1–16.
[8] J.P. Wold, K. Jorgensen, F. Lundby, Nondestructive measurement of light-induced oxidation in dairy products by fluorescence spectroscopy and imaging, J. Dairy. Sci. 85 (2002) 1693–1704.

[9] R. Bro, F. van den Berg, A. Thybo, C.M. Andersen, B.M. Jorgensen, H. Andersen, Multivariate data analysis as a tool in advanced quality monitoring in the food production chain, Trends Food Sci. Technol. 13 (2002) 235−244.
[10] K. Apperson, K.A. Leiper, I.P. Mc Keown, D.J.S. Birch, Beer fluorescence and the isolation, characterization and silica adsorption of haze-active beer proteins, J. Inst. Brew. 108 (2) (2002) 193−199.
[11] J. Christensen, A.M. Ladefoged, L. Norgaard, Rapid determination of bitterness in beer using fluorescence spectroscopy and chemometrics, J. Inst. Brew. 111 (1) (2005) 3−10.
[12] M.G. Duyvis, R. Hilhorst, C. Laane, D.J. Evans, D.J.M. Schmedding, Role of riboflavin in beer flavor instability: determination of levels of riboflavin and its origin in beer by fluorometric apoprotein titration, J. Agric. Food Chem. 50 (2002) 1548−1552.
[13] E. Sikorska, T. Gorecki, I.V. Khmelinskii, M. Sikorski, D. De Keukeleire, Analysis of Australian beers using fluorescence spectroscopy, J. Inst. Brew. 110 (2004) 267−275.
[14] E. Sikorska, et al., Chapter 19 − Fluorescence spectroscopy and imaging instruments for food quality evaluation, Evaluation Technologies for Food Quality II, Woodhead Publishing, 2019, pp. 491−533. Available from: https://doi.org/10.1016/B978-0-12-814217-2.00019-6.
[15] F. Huan, W. Hai-Long, W. Tong, L. Wan-Jun, C. An-Qi, D. Yu-Jie, et al., Excitation-emission matrix fluorescence spectroscopy coupled with multi-way chemometric techniques for characterization and classification of Chinese lager beers, Food Chem. (2020) 128235. Available from: https://doi.org/10.1016/j.foodchem.2020.128235.
[16] J.R. Lakowicz (Ed.), Principles of Fluorescence Spectroscopy., 3rd edition, Springer, New York, 2006.
[17] Valeur B., Molecular Fluorescence: Principles and Applications, Weinheim: VCH, Wiley; 2001.
[18] J. Christensen, L. Norgaard, R. Bro, S.B. Engelsen, Multivariate autofluorescence of intact food systems, Chem. Rev. 106 (6) (2006) 1979−1994.
[19] K. Kumar, M. Tarai, A.K. Mishra, Unconventional steady-state fluorescence spectroscopy as an analytical technique for analyses of complex- mutifluorophobic mixtures, Trends Anal. Chem. 97 (2017) 216−243.
[20] D. Patra, A.K. Mishra, Recent developments in multi-component synchronous fluorescence scan analysis, Trends Anal. Chem. 21 (2002) 787−798.
[21] E. Sikorska, I. Khmelinskii, M. Sikorski, Analysis of olive oils by fluorescence spectroscopy: methods and applications, in: D.D. Boskou (Ed.), Olive Oil - Constituents, Quality, Health Properties and Bioconversions, Intech Europe, Rijeka, 2012.
[22] J. Rizkallah, F.J. Morales, L. Ait-ameur, V. Fogliano, A. Hervieu, M. Courel, et al., Front face fluorescence spectroscopy and multiway analysis for process control and NFC prediction in industrially processed cookies, Chemom. Intell. Lab. Syst. 93 (2008) 99−107.
[23] K. Kumar, A.K. Mishra, Analysis of dilute aqueous multifluorophoric mixtures using excitation-emission matrix fluorescence (EEMF) and Total Synchronous Fluorescence (TSF) spectroscopy: a comparative evaluation, Talanta 117 (2013) 209−220.
[24] K. Abbas, R. Karoui, A. Ait-Kaddour, Application of synchronous xuorescence spectroscopy for the determination of some chemical parameters in PDO french blue cheeses, Eur. Food Res. Technol. 234 (2012) 457−465.
[25] J. Sadecka, J. Tothova, Fluorescence spectroscopy and chemometrics in the food classification − a review, Czech J. Food Sci. 25 (2007) 159−173.
[26] M. Bahram, R. Bro, C. Stedmon, A. Afkhami, Handling of Rayleigh and Raman scatter for PARAFAC modeling of fluorescence data using interpolation, J. Chemom. 20 (3−4) (2006) 99−105. Available from: https://doi.org/10.1002/cem.978.

[27] P.H.C. Eilers, P.M. Kroonenberg, Modeling and correction of Raman and Rayleigh scatter in fluorescence landscapes, Chemom. Intell. Lab. Syst. 130 (2014) 1–5.
[28] G.G. Guilbault, Practical Fluorescence, Marcel Dekker, New York, 1999.
[29] E. Sikorska, J. Chmielewski, J. Koziol, I.V. Khmelinskii, R. Herance, J.L. Bourdelande, et al., Photo-induced features of some lager beers. Polish, J. Food Nutr. Sci. 53 (2003) 113–118.
[30] W. Friedrich (Ed.), Vitamins, Walter de Gruyter, Berlin, New York, 1988.
[31] L.I. Nord, P. Vaag, J.O. Duus, Quantification of organic and amino acids in beer by 1H NMR spectroscopy, Anal. Chem. 76 (2004) 4790–4798.
[32] F. Shahidi, M. Naczk, In Phenolics in Food and Nutraceuticals, CRC Press, Boca Raton, FL, 2003.
[33] L.M.L. Nollet (Ed.), In Handbook of Food Analysis, Marcel Dekker, Inc, New York, 2004.
[34] A.B. Foraker, C.M. Khantwal, P.W. Swaan, Current perspectives on the cellular uptake and trafficking of riboflavin, Adv. Drug. Deliv. Rev. 55 (2003) 1467–1483.
[35] K. Huvaere, M.L. Andersen, M. Storme, J. Van Bocxlaer, L.H. Skibsted, D. De Keukeleire, Flavin-induced photodecomposition of sulfur-containing amino acids is decisive in the formation of beer lightstruck flavor, Photochem. Photobiol. Sci. 5 (2006) 961–969.
[36] A. Moller, E. Saxholt, A.T. Christensen, H.B. Hartkopp, Danish Food Composition Databank, version 5.0, Food Informatics, Inst. Food Saf. Nutrition, Dan. Veterinary Food Adm. (2002).
[37] P. Vinas, N. Balsalobre, C. Lopez-Erroz, M. Hernandez Cordoba, Liquid chromatographic analysis of riboflavin vitamers in foods using fluorescence detection, J. Agric. Food Chem. 52 (7) (2004) 1789–1794.
[38] S.D.M. Islam, T. Susdorf, A. Penzkofer, P. Hegemann, Fluorescence quenching of flavin adenine dinucleotide in aqueous solution by pH dependent isomerisation and photo-induced electron transfer, Chem. Phys. 295 (2003) 137–149.
[39] C. Andres-Lacueva, F. Mattivi, D. Tonon, Determination of riboflavin, flavin mononucleotide and flavin–adenine dinucleotide in wine and other beverages by high-performance liquid chromatography with fluorescence detection, J. Chromatogr. A 823 (1998) 355–363.
[40] T. Erbe, H. Bruckner, Chromatographic determination of amino acid enantiomers in beers and raw materials used for their manufacture, J. Chromatogr. A 881 (2000) 81–91.
[41] S. Gorinstein, A. Caspi, M. Zemser, S. Trakhtenberg, Comparative contents of some phenolics in beer, red and white wines, Nutr. Res. 20 (2000) 131–139.
[42] M. Nardini, F. Natella, C. Scaccini, A. Ghiselli, Phenolic acids from beer are absorbed and extensively metabolized in humans, J. Nutr. Biochem. 17 (2006) 14–22.
[43] D. Cho, W.L. Mattice, Quenching of the fluorescence of monomeric procyanidins by dimethyl sulfoxide, J. Phys. Chem. 94 (1990) 3847–3851.
[44] F.G. Sanchez, C. Carnero, A. Heredia, Fluorometric determination of p-coumaric acid in beer, J. Agric. Food Chem. 36 (1988) 80–82.
[45] E. Sikorska, A. Gliszczynska-Swiglo, M. Insinska-Rak, I. Khmelinskii, D. De Keukeleire, M. Sikorski, Simultaneous analysis of riboflavin and aromatic amino acids in beer using fluorescence and multivariate calibration methods, Anal. Chim. Acta 613 (2) (2008) 207–217. Available from: https://doi.org/10.1016/j.aca.2008.02.063.
[46] S. Wold, K. Esbensen, P. Geladi, Principal component analysis, Chemom. Intell. Lab. 2 (1987) 37–52.
[47] W. Wu, D.L. Massart, Regularised nearest neighbour classification method for pattern recognition of near infrared spectra, Anal. Chim. Acta 349 (1997) 253–261.

[48] Ewa Sikorska, Fluorescence spectroscopy and chemometrics in analysis of beverages, Quality Control in the Beverage Industry, Academic Press, 2019, pp. 161–203. Available from: https://doi.org/10.1016/B978-0-12-816681-9.00005-9.
[49] E. Sikorska, Beer in health and disease prevention II, F Fluorescence Methods for Analysis of Beer, Academic Press, 2009, pp. 963–976. Available from: https://doi.org/10.1016/b978-0-12-373891-2.00095-x.
[50] P.F. Heelis, The photophysical and photochemical properties of flavins (isoalloxazines), Chem. Soc. Rev. 11 (1982) 15–39.
[51] K. Huvaere, K. Olsen, M.L. Andersen, L.H. Skibsted, A. Heyerick, D. De Keukeleire, Riboflavin-sensitized photooxidation of isohumulones and derivatives, Photochem. Photobiol. Sci. 3 (2004) 337–340.
[52] M.R. Goldsmith, P.J. Rogers, N.M. Cabral, K.P. Ghiggino, F.A. Roddick, Riboflavin triplet quenchers inhibit lightstruck flavor formation in beer, J. Am. Soc. Brew. Chem. 63 (2005) 177–184.
[53] E.M. Kahle, M. Zarnkow, F. Jacob, Substances in beer that cause fluorescence: evaluating the qualitative and quantitative determination of these ingredients, Eur. Food Res. Technol. 245 (2019) 2727–2737. Available from: https://doi.org/10.1007/s00217-019-03394-x.
[54] Rasmus Bro, PARAFAC: tutorial and applications, Chemom. Intell. Lab. Syst. 38 (2) (1997) 149–171. Available from: https://doi.org/10.1016/s0169-7439(97)00032-4.
[55] K.R. Murphy, C.A. Stedmon, D. Graeber, R. Bro, Fluorescence spectroscopy and multi-way techniques. PARAFAC, Anal. Methods 5 (2013) 6557–6566.

CHAPTER FOUR

Raman spectroscopy combined with multivariate analysis in quality analysis of food and pharmaceutical materials

Seekha Naik and Monalisa Mishra
Neural Developmental Biology Lab, Department of Life Science, NIT Rourkela, Rourkela, India

4.1 Introduction

Food-borne diseases are a major concern worldwide. The Centers for Disease Control and Prevention investigated 48 million people to detect the effect of food-borne diseases on human beings. According to this report, 128,000 people get hospitalized, and 3000 people die in a year in America due to diseases associated with food [1]. Consequently, food safety is concerned to keep everyone healthy. Food products are analyzed to detect bacterial toxins, followed by biochemical analysis. These methods are easy and less expensive, less labor-consuming but time overwhelming and not applicable for all the bacteria. Commonly used methods include nucleic acid−base methods, DNA−RNA sequence amplification followed by gel detection, molecular typing, polymerase chain reaction analysis, biosensing, and next-generation sequencing. These methods cannot distinguish between live and dead bacteria. Furthermore, it varies for different food materials. Thus, a robust, less time-consuming, less expensive, accurate method is required to detect the contaminants present in the food materials. Several traditional methods like chromatographic techniques [2,3], mass spectroscopy [4], and enzyme biosensors [5] are used to ascertain the food quality. These methods are complicated, take a long time for sample preparation, and provide poor spectra. To overcome this method, hyperspectral imaging methods were developed. To overcome all these technical difficulties surface-enhanced Raman spectroscopy (SERS) was developed and used to detect the food contamination of different materials

Food Quality Analysis.
DOI: https://doi.org/10.1016/B978-0-323-95988-9.00002-3

present within the food. Raman spectroscopy is an evolving method to detect chemicals in a rapid, specific, nondestructive manner. It is often attached with high-performance liquid chromatography mass spectrometry to detect the chemicals in a more precise manner [6]. Infrared spectroscopy provides high sensitivity and easy detection. However, the sample containing water interferes with spectral imaging [7].

4.2 Principles of Raman spectroscopy

Taking the inelastic scattering method into account, Raman and Krishnan developed Raman spectroscopy in 1928 [8]. When monochromatic light of high intensity falls upon a sample, most of the photons have no energy exchange with sample molecules. The scattered photons change their direction with the same frequency as the excitation photons, and such elastic scattering is known as Rayleigh scattering. Furthermore, few scattered photons (100^{-10} to 10^{-6}) have energy exchanges with the same molecules. The direction and frequency of the scattered photons may also change. Such inelastic scattering is called Raman scattering. When scattered photons lose or gain energy, they will shift to a longer or shorter wavelength. As a result, Stokes lines and anti-Stokes lines appear as spectra. The frequency difference between Stokes scattered light and incident light is known as Raman shift. It is expressed as $\Delta\nu$ in cm^{-1}. Stokes scattering is stronger than anti-Stokes scattering and is thus used for food analysis [9].

4.3 Raman signal

During molecular vibration, the polarization change and different types of vibration are present within a sample and only a few of them give Raman signals [10]. Strong Raman signals appear due to polarization of functional groups like C–X, where X stands for F, Cl Br, and I. $C{-}NO_2$, C–S, S–S, C = C, and C = N appear in the spectrum due to change of strong polarization [10]. Strong Raman peaks that appear for melamine, urea, penicillin G, ampicillin, and lactose are assigned to plane breathing II mode. The frequency shift of scattered light is exhibited as spectral bands in the Raman spectrum. Different spectral bands have dissimilar functional or chemical bonds. Thus, Raman spectroscopy can reveal the fingerprint of specific molecules and bonds present within the samples. Consequently, Raman spectroscopy can determine the specific composition of the molecule [11].

4.4 Types of Raman spectroscopy used for food analysis

The Raman spectroscopy, in conjunction with other techniques, is commonly used for food analysis. Such techniques include (1) micro-Raman spectroscopy, (2) Raman imaging, (3) SERS, (4) near infrared Raman spectroscopy (NIRS), (5) Fourier transform Raman spectroscopy, and (5) spatial offset Raman spectroscopy (SORS). Each method for food analysis is described below.

4.4.1 Micro Raman spectroscopy

Raman spectroscopy in combination with optical microscopy is referred to as Raman microscopy. In Raman microscopy, Raman scattering is accomplished by pointing the laser light through an objective lens to the sample [12]. Raman microscopy is simple in comparison to Raman confocal microscopy concerning the pinhole. However, Raman microscopy is preferred these days due to its high contrast and resolution over an optical microscope. In confocal micro-Raman spectroscopy, a pinhole guides the light source and a splitter beam focuses it to an objective lens via diffraction to the specimen. The scattered light is collected and collimated by the same detector to the pinhole. The detector pinhole reflects the light that is out of focus and collects only the signals that are present in the same focal point.

4.4.2 Raman imaging

Raman imaging aims to visualize the distribution of the chemical composition concerning the position of the sample [12–14]. It collects the information in a two-dimensional manner, that is, from the x- and y-axis and combines this information with wavelength dimension. Thus, each information corresponds to the location for which spectral analysis has been carried out. Each pixel collected in the Raman spectrum corresponds to the spectral background measurements. The most noteworthy advantage of Raman spectroscopy is that it does not need any sample preparation [15,16]. Raman imaging can be divided into two types: point scanning imaging and wide-field imaging [17]. The first one collects the information one by one. The sample moves from one specific point to the other in a highly precise manner. In this method, the spectral resolution is very high, and it gives the full spectra. Its disadvantages are that it is time-consuming and often the laser damages the sample. This technique involves inline scanning, which means the scan takes place by laser line. The sample moves to the automated stage perpendicular to the incident laser line. The scanning is weaker than point scanning, and there is no relative movement between the laser and the sample. It is difficult to determine the spectral data.

4.4.3 Surface-enhanced Raman spectroscopy

In SERS, a confocal microscope is used in two different ways: point scanning and line scanning [18]. In this scanning, the data are collected from each point. Although the resolution is high, it often causes damage to the samples and consumes time. The inline scanning method collects the information of each line. In the Raman spectrum, each spatial location is collected in a line manner. The resolution is less in these spectra, and it is less time-consuming. However, these data are often difficult to interpret. The major drawback of Raman spectra is its scattering signal (inelastically scattered photon) is very weak. That is, one out of 106–108 photons is scattered inelastically. Consequently, if the concentration of the sample is low, then it is difficult to detect, thereby limiting its application in the food industry [19–21]. To overcome this problem, rough surface or noble metallic nanoparticles (NPs) were introduced.

This helps to enhance the RAMAN signal between 10^7 to 10^{14} times [22,23]. SERS methods are classified into two types (1) label-free or direct SERS (2) label-based SERS. In the direct SERS method, the substrate directly detects the intrinsic fingerprint. This method is simple, cost-effective, high speed, and does not interfere with other components [24–26].

4.4.4 Near-infrared Raman spectroscopy

NIRS uses the near-infrared region (from 780 to 2500 nm) to analyze the sample. It is based on molecular overtone and combination vibrations.

Both bands are found in the NIR region are very broad and result in complex spectra [27]. Thus, it is difficult to assign specific features for a particular chemical. This technique works in combination with multivariate (multiple variables) calibration techniques to deduce the chemical information. This technique was discovered by William Herschel in the 19th century [28]. The commercialization of this technique begins in 1950. In the 1980s a stand-alone NIRS system was developed for chemical analysis. In the 1990s, light fiber optics was used for the design of monochromator detectors [29].

In NIRS, there is a source, a detector, and a dispersive component. The dispersive component may be a prism used for diffraction gating to detect the intensity of different wavelengths. For wavelength above ~1000 nm, an interferometer is used [30]. A quartz halogen light is used as a source of NIR radiation. Light-emitting diodes are also used as a source of NIR radiation. For highly precise wavelength laser or frequency, combs are used as a source of radiation. For the short NIR range, silicon-based CCDs (charge-coupled device) are used [31]. However, they are not sensitive over 100 nm. InGaAs and PbS can provide high quantum efficiency for wavelengths more than 1100 nm [32]. Both silicon-based and InGaAs are combined in a single instrument to detect ultraviolet (UV)—visible and NIR spectra simultaneously. NIRS for chemical imaging uses a 2D array detector with an acoustic optic tunable filter [33].

4.4.5 Fourier transform Raman spectroscopy

The Fourier transform Raman spectroscopy uses a similar principle as Fourier transform infrared (FTIR) spectroscopy. In this instrument, a YAG: Nd^{3+} laser (1064 nm) is used to excite the sample [34]. The excitation energy used is lower than the absorption band energies of organic systems. Afterward, the fluorescence is minimized. This instrument is associated either with a microscope or optical fiber to scan the surface area of a few micrometer squares [35]. The scanning facilitates the Raman mapping. The use of interferometric spectroscopy has a limited result. The work is carried out with analog computers, but it can be replaced with digital computers. This method is relatively easy and compatible with personal computers. Thus, for commercialization, the development of computer-controlled spectrometers is essential for rapid acquiring, computing, and displaying high-quality and high-resolution spectra. Recently, fiber optics have been used in Raman spectroscopy [36]. Fiber optics, integrated optics, and micro-optics in combination with laser expand the analytical ability of Raman spectroscopy. With fiber optic probes, high-temperature process streams and hazardous sampling are possible [37].

4.4.6 Spatial offset Raman spectroscopy

The concept of SORS lies in a point-like illumination of the sample surface. The SORS collection efficiency can be improved by integrating the signals present in the circle, that is, the illumination point. An SORS having biomedical applications has ring illumination [38]. The signal is collected from the ring using optical fibers. The spatial offset is facilitated by the radius of the illumination. Using a conical lens (axicon), a ring-shaped profile of the laser beam is generated. With axicon, the ring diameter and ring thickness can be altered. With the large ring, the radius resulted in large illumination [39]. Thus, the increase of the illumination of laser power for larger spatial offsets is beneficial for in vivo applications. SORS gets the benefit from the accuracy of measurement and enhances penetration depths [40]. The use of light in modulating SORS imaging is facilitated by micro-electro-mechanical systems. SORS measurements are performed at 785, 808 and 830 nm [39]. SORS interferes with tissue with more pigmentation or dark in color.

4.4.7 Raman spectral analysis

The Raman spectra are multifarious and hence require proper analysis to elucidate the detailed information about the sample that is not visible to naked eyes. Henceforth, the Raman spectra are processed and analyzed to derive the information that is not visible to the naked eye [41,42]. While processing data, noise, artifacts, and unnecessary signals are removed from the raw data generated by the equipment [42]. Data processing includes intensity calibration, wavenumber calibration, normalization, background correction, and dimension reduction [43]. While selecting data processing approach, different methods are used to avoid data loss [44,45]. Multivariate analysis extracts different data from Raman spectra using chemometrics to classify and distinguish the sample. These methods are further classified into unsupervised and supervised pattern recognition methods. Unsupervised models detect the signal from the hidden structure and unlabeled data, which reduces the spectral dimension. Principle component analysis (PCA) is a widely used unsupervised learning algorithm [46,47]. For better classification of unknown samples, it is further combined with clustering algorithms. Instead of supervised pattern recognition, a series of known samples are used for mathematical calculation. Some of the widely used techniques include artificial neural networks, linear discriminant analysis, partial least square (PLS) discrimination analysis, and support vector machine [48,49]. The prediction model recognizes the connection and stimulus of the variables and uses this information to predict a parameter for new observation. Since the selection of an appropriate mathematical model is crucial, several models have been proposed and utilized for the evaluation of results.

4.5 Raman spectroscopy to detect the hazards caused by biological agents

Microbes grow on food and can cause contamination of food and spread diseases [50,51]. Examples of microbes that can cause adulteration of food include bacteria, viruses, fungi, and many parasites. Food-borne viruses include rotavirus, norovirus, astrovirus, and Hepatitis A. Bacteria responsible for food illness include *Staphylococcus*, *Salmonella*, *Listeria*, *Vibrio*, *Bacillus*, Shiga-toxigenic *Escherichia coli*. Micro-Raman spectroscopy can detect food contamination at different stages [52,53]. Raman spectra can distinguish many strains of *Staphylococcus* [52,53]. Acetobacter species were identified with 5%–99% accuracy by using Raman spectroscopy connected to a neural network [54]. Dispersive Raman spectroscopy can reveal strains like *E. coli*, *Pseudomonas*, and *Bacillus* [55]. Confocal Raman spectroscopy can distinguish between 23 strains with 87.5%–95.8% accuracy [56]. Food-borne bacterial biofilm can be detected using Raman microscopy [57,58]. The Raman peak obtained is directly correlated with the amount of biofilm. Raman microscopy can distinguish the planktonic form from the microbial biofilm. Raman spectra can distinguish the peak of viable but nonculturable bacteria (VBNC) [59,60]. D_2O-labeled confocal Raman microscopy can distinguish the dead cells of VBNC bacteria in water. The chemometric method can distinguish six *Listeria* species using Raman PLS analysis. Raman microscopy can detect the steak surface to count the lactic acid bacteria present in beef during packaging [61]. Water-borne pathogens are detected by Raman spectroscopy and SERS. The former can detect the alteration of amino acid and protein content in spoiled food over time [62]. Norovirus can be detected using Raman spectroscopy method [63]. Pear juice was placed over SERS and detected by Raman mapping. A correlation between *Alternaria alternata* Raman intensity and fungal concentration was detected [64]. Raman analysis along with nanostructures is described elaborately in the nanostructure section.

4.6 Multivariate analysis

Raman spectroscopy with NIR excitation coupled with multivariate analysis is useful for various studies. A multivariate algorithm is used to analyze the zearalenone content of ground maize in a single-step analysis. Raman spectra were collected in a multivariate analysis. The detected zearalenone concentration ranges from 6.9–800.2 μg/kg of aflatoxins [65].

4.7 Raman spectroscopy for detection of food

Raman spectroscopy is widely used for the detection of both animal and plant products used for food [11,66]. Raman spectra of different meats concerning the handling, processing, and storage are available [67]. Raman spectroscopy of different plant substances and quality parameters have been reviewed [68]. It is widely used for the detection of plant species due to its rapid and nondestructive properties [68]. In Raman spectroscopy, sample preparation is not required, and all measurements are done using fiber optics. The effect of water on Raman spectra is negligible. Thus Raman spectroscopy is used to detect the quality of food [69,70]. Many studies analyze the oils and fats under Raman microscopy [71,72]. The content of fatty acid in milk was analyzed using Raman spectroscopy [73]. A Raman spectrum was used for the detection of unsaturated fatty acid in salmons [74]. Fourier transform Raman spectroscopy has been used for the detection of amino acid content in the protein of meat samples [71].

4.7.1 Raman for milk analysis

Since milk is a matrix, sample preparation is needed for this. Raman spectroscopy data may be affected by the big molecules present within the milk like protein and fat. Hence, separation or pretreatment is required for sample preparation. To eliminate the cosmic spikes, techniques like robust summation, upper bound spectrum, filtering techniques, and nearest neighbor comparison are used [75]. Polynomial fitting, air PLS, and wavelength transformation are used as an algorithm to correct the baseline. Normalization algorithms are employed for evaluating the real samples. Raman spectroscopy has been used in many kinds of studies [76–78]. Raman microscopy can help to detect the parameters like lactose, fats, fatty acid, and proteins quantitatively while analyzing the samples. Ultraviolet resonance Raman spectroscopy has been used for qualitative analysis of the milk sample. This analysis helps to determine the chromophores like aromatic amino acid, nucleic acid, and lipid present within the milk bacteria [79]. Bacteria having minor differences were not analyzed by this technique. This method still uses traditional colony counting while plating the bacteria. Recently, SERS has been used along with chemometrics for the analysis of food.

4.7.2 Raman spectroscopy for butter and margarine

Butter and margarine are fats dispersed in water. Margarine is a saturated vegetable oil, whereas butter is obtained from animals. Henceforth, butter is costlier than margarine. The adulteration of butter is often done by adding margarine into it. The chemometric method along with Raman analysis gives various ways to analyze the adulteration of fat of butter [80]. Raman spectroscopy is also combined with PLS and artificial neural networks (ANNs) to make it simple. ANNs can distinguish the variation between the butter qualities obtained in different seasons. It takes only a few seconds with ANNs to detect the quality of butter with less time for sample preparation. Uysal et al. successfully employed Raman spectroscopy to detect the adulteration of butter with margarine [81].

4.7.3 Raman spectroscopy for yogurt

Protein adulteration in yogurt can be detected using Raman spectroscopy. In yogurt, a fast green method is adopted to determine the adulteration of yogurt. Yogurts are often found to blend with fat or vegetable oil. Raman spectroscopy coupled with PCA was used to analyze yogurt. Temperature also has some effect on Raman spectra. Fermentation and yogurt processing affects the composition of the yogurt. Using NIR and chemometrics methods, adulteration of yogurt was determined [82].

A total of 197 types of adulterated yogurt samples were detected by Xu et al. [83], who detected gelatin powder and soya powder in yogurt.

4.7.4 Raman spectroscopy for meat analysis

Over time, it has become a demand to know the origin of meat. Meat cannot be easily contaminated as it is sold in its solid form. In this context, minced meat or meat fillings are easy to be adulterated [84]. Turkey leg was analyzed to detect the flavor and quality of the leg. Peaks for tenderness and juiciness were also analyzed using Raman spectroscopy.

4.7.5 Raman for olive oil

Olive oil is enriched with fatty acids, vitamins, and pigments. Its hydrolysis resulted in free fatty acid (FFA) and residues of glycerol. The presence of FFA helps to determine the shelf-life and flavor of the olive oil. Many factors stimulate the formation of FFA in olive oil [85,86]. Thus, FFA is regarded as one of the parameters to measure the quality of the oil. Olive oil with more than 3.3% FFA is unsuitable for consumption and hence needs to be refined prior to the consumption. FTIR is used to determine the FFA in olive oil. Raman spectroscopy can determine the FFA less than 0.1% [87].

4.7.6 Raman spectroscopy for beverages

Carbohydrates are the main source of metabolism. Still, higher consumption of carbohydrates result in metabolic disorder. Taking this information into account, carbohydrate level was analyzed in soft drinks. Raman spectroscopy was employed to ascertain the amount of mono- and disaccharide in soft drinks [88]. The water content of the beverages does not interfere with Raman scattering. The PLS analysis was used to get the calibration curve and kinetic study of the beverages of the analysis using Raman spectroscopy [89]. The choice of proper spectral change and a number of variables were employed in this model. In soft drinks, the main peaks were obtained for glucose, sucrose, and fructose. The glucose bands appeared at 517, 849, 913, and 1124 cm^{-1}. For fructose, the bands appeared at 627, 707, 870, 819, and 1071 cm^{-1}. Bands at 745 and 796 cm^{-1} were found to be specific for sucrose molecules. Along with sugar, aroma peaks have also been determined using Raman spectroscopy. For aromatized soda, aroma, and citric acid, the aroma has no distinct peaks. Raman analysis takes only 30 s, which is lesser than the chemical and enzymatic methods [89,90].

4.7.7 Wine analysis

The formation of wine is a two-step process. The first step involves the development of a sugar-rich solution by adding yeast. Yeast consumes sugar to produce alcohol. These steps can be easily determined by MarqMetrix all in one Raman system [91]. The ratios of sugar to alcohol determine the sweetness of the alcohols. Several components responsible for the flavor can be determined by using this technique. MarqMetrix gives the sample in both solid and liquid items. Wine can be analyzed efficiently using Raman spectroscopy [92,93].

4.8 Detection of chemicals using Raman analysis

Raman spectroscopy is a robust method to analyze the chemicals within the food [6,94]. Mycotoxin's toxicity for human health was detected by Raman spectroscopy. A total of 0.5–15 μg/kg of aflatoxins was detected in nuts, grains, and dried figs. Spoiled meat can be detected from within the packet by using Raman spectroscopy. Raman spectra can detect the planktonic form and biofilm formation stage in the food. Detection of fungi by SERS causes a threat to public health. Mycotoxins are produced by the fungi and cause immune deficiency and cancer. Aflatoxin is determined in nuts, grains, figs, and milk. Raman spectroscopy can detect SERS intensity with an $R^2 = 0.9958$ [95]. Bisphenol A, a common chemical used in plastic, was detected using SERS. SERS on a flower-like silver-based coupled with multivariate analysis can detect the coumarin to a certain extent. Raman spectral imaging can detect potassium bromide in all-purpose flour. Raman spectroscopy can detect melamine in milk. SERS was analyzed to be detected using Raman microscope. Raman microscopy can detect adulteration of olive oil, glucose, fructose, malt, butter with margarine and pistachio, and green peas [96–98].

4.9 Raman detection for pharmaceuticals

Raman spectra have an advantage over other estimated methods for detecting the chemical composition of pharmaceutical materials. It includes

(1) choice of exciting wavelength, (2) easy accumulation of scattered signals, (3) effective and reproducible enhancement, and (4) easy handling of substrates. Typically, a drug consists of active agents, binders, and additives. Raman imaging enables to distinguish different percentages of composition within the drug in a time- and cost-saving manner [99–102]. The chemical composition of the packaging material of capsules was analyzed by Eliasson and Matousek using Raman spectroscopy [103,104]. Several polymeric materials used for drug delivery were analyzed using SORS [105]. SORS signals of the drugs were analyzed using gold NPs. Raman spectroscopy can analyze Chinese medicines [106]. Thalidomide was detected by micro-Raman in chick embryos [107]. The results showed relative Raman intensity variations of vasculatures for some characteristic peaks. SERS can detect the antibiotics (enrofloxacin, ciprofloxacin, and chloramphenicol) amount in food and drug [108,109] using silver nanostructures. Antitumor compounds (Ptcoordinate) with DNA were detected by Smulevich et al. [110]. Abuse of amphetamine and methamphetamine was detected by Sulk et al. [111].

4.10 Raman to detect nanomaterials

Raman microscopy can visualize the internal structure without any further labeling. Kneipp and coworkers used gold colloids to know the chemical composition of the cell [112–114]. They proposed a nanosensor to detect the Raman signature [115]. SERS microspectroscopy with a silver hydrosol allows studying doxorubicin complexes in cancer cells. SERS spectra of doxorubicin and other biomolecules adsorbed on silver island films were also observed [116]. Raman microspectrometer was used to detect the live tumors of mice using single-walled carbon nanotubes (SWCNT) or arginine–glycine–aspartic acid peptide modified SWCNT [117]. Raman spectroscopy enables CNT localization to target tumors in several colors using preclinical studies. Near-field SERS used to label single dye molecules and dye-labeled DNA with a 100 nm [118,119]. Bionanomaterials are ideal in diagnosis for drug delivery. Various metal NPs are used for SERS imaging. One of the ways to incorporate NPs in living cells is by incubating them with colloidal metal [120]. Electroporation is also used to incorporate metals [121,122]. The third way of incorporation is by reduction of metals [123]. This method used Ag ions to deposit on the cell surface. Optic fiber nanoprobes are used to get inside the cell. Nguyen et al. functionalized AuNPs to detect SERS [124–126]. In AuNP, Au is present in the core and covered with a malachite green isothiocyanate. The image targets dye and polyethylene glycol. Nonbinding negative controls NP without any antibody attachment. AuNPs functionalized with an anti-CD19 antibody have specific markers. Raman spectroscopy has been used to visualize deep tissue in live animals. *E. coli* and *Staphylococcus epidermis* were detected in label-free SERS mapping using AgNPs [127]. Ag-coated magnetic NPs can detect *Acinetobacter baylyi* and *E. coli* using SERS. SERS spectra of pathogens captured polycarbonate membrane. Bacteria can be detected using this technique. Magnetic NPs were used to detect *E. coli*. The bacteria cell concentration was detected as 10^2 CFU/mL with 4% accuracy. SERS microscopy along with AgNPs and PCA can detect the *Listeria monocytogenes* in ham, *Salmonella* in eggs, and *Salmonella* in smoked salmon [128]. Au nanorod can distinguish SERS method to detect the fungi with an accuracy of 98.31% [129]. *A. alternata* was detected by using Ag nanodots array [64].

4.11 Raman analysis to prevent physical hazards

Often the food and pharmaceutical compounds are mixed with superfluous materials like metals, plastics, rocks, woods, and plastics while processing and packing. These superfluous materials are sharp, hard, and may cause mechanical damage while consuming that food material [130,131]. Various hand-picked methods like sieves and visual perceptions are used to separate them. In offices, spectroscopy and thermal techniques are used for the analysis of plastic, another superfluous material. Identification of plastic is easy due to its size, shape, and chemical composition [132]. Recently, Raman spectroscopy was used for the analysis of five different plastics from the atmosphere by using stimulated Raman scattering (SRS) microscopy [133]. Using SRS microscopy, 88 microplastics were detected. The contamination of microplastics in tap and environmental water was detected [132]. Plastic size of 100 nm to 10 μm was detected using the SERS method [134]. Micro-Raman spectroscopy detects microplastics in the white wines cap stopper. To date, only a few analyses have been carried out using Raman spectroscopy to prevent physical or mechanical damage by the extraneous materials. The successful analysis by means of Raman spectroscopy suggests its wide application in detecting the extraneous materials present in several substances. Although the data obtained from Raman spectroscopy are very promising, only a handful of analyses were carried out using this technique. All these results suggest Raman spectroscopy can be used as a robust tool in the future to avoid mechanical damage to food materials.

4.12 Future perspective

Raman spectroscopy is widely used to detect toxic or inedible substances within the food. However, only limited laboratories use this method due to challenges coming across with this technique. One of the major challenges is the reference sample or the database, which is confined only to a particular group. Raman spectra are used for the analysis of different samples that are prepared by using various techniques. As a consequence, a complete worldwide database is in need for complete analysis of the samples. Such a database will work as a reference for the analysis of any sample. Raman along with multivariate analysis can be used for the separation of the components present within the sample. Integrated sensors should be developed to detect the chemical composition of the food. An automated chemical detection method is required to detect the chemical composition of the food materials. The other challenges in SERS are the inhomogeneous distribution of hot spot detection. The inhomogeneous detection resulted in variation in the sample analysis. The major shortcoming of this method is that it cannot distinguish the dead bacterial biofilm from the live bacteria. Advanced chemometrics and machine learning techniques can be combined for the detection of the safety and surveillance of food. With the worldwide database and sample preparation, Raman spectroscopy can be used as an indispensable tool to detect the biological, chemical, and physical hazardous substances present within the food.

Acknowledgments

MM lab is supported by the Department of Biotechnology, Ministry of Science and Technology [SERB/EMR/2017/003054, BT/PR21857/NNT/28/1238/2017, and Odisha DBT 3325/ST(BIO)-02/2017] for financial assistance.

References

[1] J.W.-F. Law, N.-S. Ab Mutalib, K.-G. Chan, L.-H. Lee, Rapid methods for the detection of foodborne bacterial pathogens: principles, applications, advantages and limitations, Front. Microbiol. 5 (2015) 770.

[2] J. Dominguez-Alvarez, M. Mateos-Vivas, D. García-Gómez, E. Rodríguez-Gonzalo, R. Carabias-Martínez, Capillary electrophoresis coupled to mass spectrometry for the determination of anthelmintic benzimidazoles in eggs using a QuEChERS with preconcentration as sample treatment, J. Chromatogr. A 1278 (2013) 166–174.

[3] P. Manzi, L. Pizzoferrato, HPLC determination of lactulose in heat treated milk, Food Bioprocess. Technol. 6 (2013) 851–857.

[4] C. Soukoulis, L. Cappellin, E. Aprea, F. Costa, R. Viola, T.D. Märk, et al., PTR-ToF-MS, a novel, rapid, high sensitivity and non-invasive tool to monitor volatile compound release during fruit post-harvest storage: the case study of apple ripening, Food Bioprocess. Technol. 6 (2013) 2831–2843.

[5] D. Alexandre, A. Melo, R. Furtado, M. Borges, E. Figueiredo, A. Biswas, et al., A rapid and specific biosensor for Salmonella typhimurium detection in milk, Food Bioprocess. Technol. 11 (2018) 748–756.

[6] H. Dies, M. Siampani, C. Escobedo, A. Docoslis, Direct detection of toxic contaminants in minimally processed food products using dendritic surface-enhanced Raman scattering substrates, Sensors 18 (2018) 2726.

[7] M. Diem, A. Mazur, K. Lenau, J. Schubert, B. Bird, M. Miljković, et al., Molecular pathology via IR and Raman spectral imaging, J. Biophotonics 6 (2013) 855–886.

[8] C.V. Raman, K.S. Krishnan, A new type of secondary radiation, Nature 121 (1928) 501–502.

[9] C.H. Camp JR, M.T. Cicerone, Chemically sensitive bioimaging with coherent Raman scattering, Nat. Photonics 9 (2015) 295–305.

[10] R. Dijkstra, F. Ariese, C. Gooijer, U.T. Brinkman, Raman spectroscopy as a detection method for liquid-separation techniques, TrAC. Trends Anal. Chem. 24 (2005) 304–323.

[11] D. Yang, Y. Ying, Applications of Raman spectroscopy in agricultural products and food analysis: a review, Appl. Spectrosc. Rev. 46 (2011) 539–560.

[12] A. Zumbusch, G.R. Holtom, X.S. Xie, Three-dimensional vibrational imaging by coherent anti-Stokes Raman scattering, Phys. Rev. Lett. 82 (1999) 4142.

[13] D. Zhang, P. Wang, M.N. Slipchenko, D. Ben-Amotz, A.M. Weiner, J.-X. Cheng, Quantitative vibrational imaging by hyperspectral stimulated Raman scattering microscopy and multivariate curve resolution analysis, Anal. Chem. 85 (2013) 98–106.

[14] N. Hayazawa, Y. Inouye, Z. Sekkat, S. Kawata, Metallized tip amplification of near-field Raman scattering, Opt. Commun. 183 (2000) 333–336.

[15] T. Vankeirsbilck, A. Vercauteren, W. Baeyens, G. Van Der Weken, F. Verpoort, G. Vergote, et al., Applications of Raman spectroscopy in pharmaceutical analysis, TrAC Trends Anal. Chem. 21 (2002) 869–877.

[16] H. Vašková, A powerful tool for material identification: Raman spectroscopy, Int. J. Math. Model. Methods Appl. Sci. 5 (2011) 1205–1212.

[17] M.D. Schaeberle, H.R. Morris, J.F.T. Ii, P.J. Treado, Peer reviewed: Raman chemical imaging spectroscopy, Anal. Chem. 71 (1999) 175A–181A.

[18] J. Fredrich, 3D imaging of porous media using laser scanning confocal microscopy with application to microscale transport processes, Phys. Chem. Earth Part. A: Solid. Earth Geodesy 24 (1999) 551–561.

[19] E. Smith, G. Dent, Modern Raman Spectroscopy: A Practical Approach, John Wiley & Sons, 2019.

[20] S. Stöckel, J. Kirchhoff, U. Neugebauer, P. Rösch, J. Popp, The application of Raman spectroscopy for the detection and identification of microorganisms, J. Raman Spectrosc. 47 (2016) 89–109.
[21] J. Zheng, L. He, Surface-enhanced Raman spectroscopy for the chemical analysis of food, Compr. Rev. Food Sci. food Saf. 13 (2014) 317–328.
[22] P.J. Goulet, D.S. Dos Santos, R.A. Alvarez-Puebla, O.N. Oliveira, R.F. Aroca, Surface-enhanced Raman scattering on dendrimer/metallic nanoparticle layer-by-layer film substrates, Langmuir 21 (2005) 5576–5581.
[23] F. Le, D.W. Brandl, Y.A. Urzhumov, H. Wang, J. Kundu, N.J. Halas, et al., Metallic nanoparticle arrays: a common substrate for both surface-enhanced Raman scattering and surface-enhanced infrared absorption, ACS Nano 2 (2008) 707–718.
[24] W. Xie, S. Schlücker, Medical applications of surface-enhanced Raman scattering, Phys. Chem. Chem. Phys. 15 (2013) 5329–5344.
[25] Z. Chen, S.M. Tabakman, A.P. Goodwin, M.G. Kattah, D. Daranciang, X. Wang, et al., Protein microarrays with carbon nanotubes as multicolor Raman labels, Nat. Biotechnol. 26 (2008) 1285–1292.
[26] L. Fabris, Gold-based SERS tags for biomedical imaging, J. Opt. 17 (2015) 114002.
[27] T. Korsman, I. Renberg, E. Dåbakk, M.B. Nilsson, Near-infrared spectrometry (NIRS) in palaeolimnology, Tracking Environmental Change Using Lake Sediments, Springer, 2002.
[28] M. Jackson, M.G. Sowa, H.H. Mantsch, Infrared spectroscopy: a new frontier in medicine, Biophys. Chem. 68 (1997) 109–125.
[29] W. Wang, J. Paliwal, Near-infrared spectroscopy and imaging in food quality and safety, Sens. Instrum. Food Qual. Saf. 1 (2007) 193–207.
[30] J.M. Amigo, S. Grassi, Configuration of hyperspectral and multispectral imaging systems, Data Handling in Science and Technology, Elsevier, 2020.
[31] M. Althobaiti, I. Al-Naib, Recent developments in instrumentation of functional near-infrared spectroscopy systems, Appl. Sci. 10 (2020) 6522.
[32] P.E. Malinowski, E. Georgitzikis, J. Maes, I. Vamvaka, F. Frazzica, J. Van Olmen, et al., Thin-film quantum dot photodiode for monolithic infrared image sensors, Sensors 17 (2017) 2867.
[33] P.J. Treado, I.W. Levin, E.N. Lewis, Indium antimonide (InSb) focal plane array (FPA) detection for near-infrared imaging microscopy, Appl. Spectrosc. 48 (1994) 607–615.
[34] U.P. Agarwal, 1064 nm FT-Raman spectroscopy for investigations of plant cell walls and other biomass materials, Front. Plant. Sci. 5 (2014) 490.
[35] R. Bhartia, L.W. Beegle, L. Deflores, W. Abbey, J. Razzell Hollis, K. Uckert, et al., Perseverance's scanning habitable environments with Raman and luminescence for organics and chemicals (SHERLOC) investigation, Space Sci. Rev. 217 (2021) 1–115.
[36] E.N. Lewis, P.J. Treado, R.C. Reeder, G.M. Story, A.E. Dowrey, C. Marcott, et al., Fourier transform spectroscopic imaging using an infrared focal-plane array detector, Anal. Chem. 67 (1995) 3377–3381.
[37] C.P. Bacon, Y. Mattley, R. Defrece, Miniature spectroscopic instrumentation: applications to biology and chemistry, Rev. Sci. Instrum. 75 (2004) 1–16.
[38] M. Abdolrazzaghi, N. Katchinskiy, A.Y. Elezzabi, P.E. Light, M. Daneshmand, Noninvasive glucose sensing in aqueous solutions using an active split-ring resonator, IEEE Sens. J. 21 (2021) 18742–18755.
[39] F. Nicolson, M.F. Kircher, N. Stone, P. Matousek, Spatially offset Raman spectroscopy for biomedical applications, Chem. Soc. Rev. 50 (2021) 556–568.
[40] F. Nicolson, B. Andreiuk, C. Andreou, H.-T. Hsu, S. Rudder, M.F. Kircher, Non-invasive in vivo imaging of cancer using surface-enhanced spatially offset Raman spectroscopy (SESORS), Theranostics 9 (2019) 5899.

[41] K. Venkatakrishna, J. Kurien, K.M. Pai, M. Valiathan, N.N. Kumar, C. Murali Krishna, et al., Optical pathology of oral tissue: a Raman spectroscopy diagnostic method, Curr. Sci. 80 (2001) 665–669.
[42] H.J. Butler, L. Ashton, B. Bird, G. Cinque, K. Curtis, J. Dorney, et al., Using Raman spectroscopy to characterize biological materials, Nat. Protoc. 11 (2016) 664–687.
[43] O. Ryabchykov, S. Guo, T. Bocklitz, Analyzing Raman spectroscopic data, Phys. Sci. Rev. (2019) 4.
[44] P. Mobili, A. Londero, G. De Antoni, A. Gomez-Zavaglia, C. Araujo-Andrade, H. Avila-Donoso, et al., Multivariate analysis of Raman spectra applied to microbiology: Discrimination of microorganisms at the species level, Rev. Mex. Fís. 56 (2010) 378–385.
[45] I. Notingher, G. Jell, P.L. Notingher, I. Bisson, O. Tsigkou, J.M. Polak, et al., Multivariate analysis of Raman spectra for in vitro non-invasive studies of living cells, J. Mol. Struct. 744 (2005) 179–185.
[46] R. Ullah, S. Khan, I.I. Chaudhary, S. Shahzad, H. Ali, M. Bilal, Cost effective and efficient screening of tuberculosis disease with Raman spectroscopy and machine learning algorithms, Photodiagn. Photodyn. Ther. 32 (2020) 101963.
[47] C. Hu, J. Wang, C. Zheng, S. Xu, H. Zhang, Y. Liang, et al., Raman spectra exploring breast tissues: comparison of principal component analysis and support vector machine-recursive feature elimination, Med. Phys. 40 (2013) 063501.
[48] N. Marigheto, E. Kemsley, M. Defernez, R. Wilson, A comparison of mid-infrared and Raman spectroscopies for the authentication of edible oils, J. Am. Oil Chem. Soc. 75 (1998) 987–992.
[49] H.M. Monavar, N. Afseth, J. Lozano, R. Alimardani, M. Omid, J. Wold, Determining quality of caviar from Caspian Sea based on Raman spectroscopy and using artificial neural networks, Talanta 111 (2013) 98–104.
[50] R. Tauxe, H. Kruse, C. Hedberg, M. Potter, J. Madden, K. Wachsmuth, Microbial hazards and emerging issues associated with produce a preliminary report to the national advisory committee on microbiologic criteria for foods, J. Food Prot. 60 (1997) 1400–1408.
[51] N.J. Ashbolt, Microbial contamination of drinking water and disease outcomes in developing regions, Toxicology 198 (2004) 229–238.
[52] K. Rebrošová, M. Šiler, O. Samek, F. Růžička, S. Bernatová, V. Holá, et al., Rapid identification of staphylococci by Raman spectroscopy, Sci. Rep. 7 (2017) 1–8.
[53] K. Rebrošová, M. Šiler, O. Samek, F. R° Užïcka, S. Bernatová, V. Holá, et al., Rapid Identification of Staphylococci by Raman spectroscopy, Sci. Rep. 7 (2017) 14846.
[54] K. Wang, L. Chen, X. Ma, L. Ma, K.C. Chou, Y. Cao, et al., Arcobacter identification and species determination using Raman spectroscopy combined with neural networks, Appl. Environ. Microbiol. 86 (2020). e00924-20.
[55] S. Jaafreh, O. Valler, J. Kreyenschmidt, K. Günther, P. Kaul, In vitro discrimination and classification of Microbial Flora of Poultry using two dispersive Raman spectrometers (microscope and Portable Fiber-Optic systems) in tandem with chemometric analysis, Talanta 202 (2019) 411–425.
[56] S. Yan, S. Wang, J. Qiu, M. Li, D. Li, D. Xu, et al., Raman spectroscopy combined with machine learning for rapid detection of food-borne pathogens at the single-cell level, Talanta 226 (2021) 122195.
[57] S.S. Rad, A.M. Sani, S. Mohseni, Biosynthesis, characterization and antimicrobial activities of zinc oxide nanoparticles from leaf extract of Mentha pulegium (L.), Microb. Pathog. 131 (2019) 239–245.
[58] S. Bujok, J. Peter, M. Halecký, P. Ecorchard, A. Machálková, G.S. Medeiros, et al., Sustainable microwave synthesis of biodegradable active packaging films based on

polycaprolactone and layered ZnO nanoparticles, Polym. Degrad. Stab. 190 (2021) 109625.
[59] L. Guo, K. Wan, J. Zhu, C. Ye, K. Chabi, X. Yu, Detection and distribution of vbnc/viable pathogenic bacteria in full-scale drinking water treatment plants, J. Hazard. Mater. 406 (2021) 124335.
[60] L. Guo, C. Ye, L. Cui, K. Wan, S. Chen, S. Zhang, et al., Population and single cell metabolic activity of UV-induced VBNC bacteria determined by CTC-FCM and D2O-labeled Raman spectroscopy, Environ. Int. 130 (2019) 104883.
[61] H. Yang, D.L. Hopkins, Y. Zhang, L. Zhu, P. Dong, X. Wang, et al., Preliminary investigation of the use of Raman spectroscopy to predict beef spoilage in different types of packaging, Meat Sci. 165 (2020) 108136.
[62] A. Zając, L. Dymińska, J. Lorenc, J. Hanuza, Fourier transform infrared and raman spectroscopy studies of the time-dependent changes in chicken meat as a tool for recording spoilage processes, Food Anal. Methods 10 (2017) 640–648.
[63] O.J. Achadu, F. Abe, T. Suzuki, E.Y. Park, Molybdenum trioxide nanocubes aligned on a graphene oxide substrate for the detection of norovirus by surface-enhanced raman scattering, ACS Appl. Mater. Interfaces 12 (2020) 43522–43534.
[64] T.-T. Pan, D.-W. Sun, H. Pu, Q. Wei, W. Xiao, Q.-J. Wang, Detection of A. alternata from pear juice using surface-enhanced Raman spectroscopy based silver nanodots array, J. Food Eng. 215 (2017) 147–155.
[65] Z. Guo, M. Wang, J. Wu, F. Tao, Q. Chen, Q. Wang, et al., Quantitative assessment of zearalenone in maize using multivariate algorithms coupled to Raman spectroscopy, Food Chem. 286 (2019) 282–288.
[66] M.-L. Xu, Y. Gao, X.X. Han, B. Zhao, Detection of pesticide residues in food using surface-enhanced Raman spectroscopy: a review, J. Agric. Food Chem. 65 (2017) 6719–6726.
[67] A.M. Herrero, Raman spectroscopy a promising technique for quality assessment of meat and fish: a review, Food Chem. 107 (2008) 1642–1651.
[68] H. Schulz, M. Baranska, Identification and quantification of valuable plant substances by IR and Raman spectroscopy, Vib. Spectrosc. 43 (2007) 13–25.
[69] R.J. Beattie, S.J. Bell, L.J. Farmer, B.W. Moss, D. Patterson, Preliminary investigation of the application of Raman spectroscopy to the prediction of the sensory quality of beef silverside, Meat Sci. 66 (2004) 903–913.
[70] S. Lohumi, S. Lee, H. Lee, B.-K. Cho, A review of vibrational spectroscopic techniques for the detection of food authenticity and adulteration, Trends Food Sci. Technol. 46 (2015) 85–98.
[71] A. Zając, J. Hanuza, L. Dymińska, Raman spectroscopy in determination of horse meat content in the mixture with other meats, Food Chem. 156 (2014) 333–338.
[72] E.F. Olsen, E.-O. Rukke, A. Flåtten, T. Isaksson, Quantitative determination of saturated-, monounsaturated-and polyunsaturated fatty acids in pork adipose tissue with non-destructive Raman spectroscopy, Meat Sci. 76 (2007) 628–634.
[73] M. Meurens, V. Baeten, S.H. Yan, E. Mignolet, Y. Larondelle, Determination of the conjugated linoleic acids in cow's milk fat by Fourier transform Raman spectroscopy, J. Agric. Food Chem. 53 (2005) 5831–5835.
[74] N.K. Afseth, J.P. Wold, V.H. Segtnan, The potential of Raman spectroscopy for characterisation of the fatty acid unsaturation of salmon, Anal. Chim. Acta 572 (2006) 85–92.
[75] L. Zhang, M.J. Henson, A practical algorithm to remove cosmic spikes in Raman imaging data for pharmaceutical applications, Appl. Spectrosc. 61 (2007) 1015–1020.
[76] J. Qin, M.S. Kim, K. Chao, S. Dhakal, B.-K. Cho, S. Lohumi, et al., Advances in Raman spectroscopy and imaging techniques for quality and safety inspection of horticultural products, Postharvest Biol. Technol. 149 (2019) 101–117.

[77] R. Joshi, S. Lohumi, R. Joshi, M.S. Kim, J. Qin, I. Baek, et al., Raman spectral analysis for non-invasive detection of external and internal parameters of fake eggs, Sens. Actuators B: Chem. 303 (2020) 127243.
[78] S. Lohumi, M.S. Kim, J. Qin, B.-K. Cho, Raman imaging from microscopy to macroscopy: quality and safety control of biological materials, TrAC Trends Anal. Chem. 93 (2017) 183–198.
[79] E.C. López-Díez, R. Goodacre, Characterization of microorganisms using UV resonance Raman spectroscopy and chemometrics, Anal. Chem. 76 (2004) 585–591.
[80] S. Lohumi, H. Lee, M.S. Kim, J. Qin, B.-K. Cho, Through-packaging analysis of butter adulteration using line-scan spatially offset Raman spectroscopy, Anal. Bioanal. Chem. 410 (2018) 5663–5673.
[81] R.S. Uysal, I.H. Boyaci, H.E. Genis, U. Tamer, Determination of butter adulteration with margarine using Raman spectroscopy, Food Chem. 141 (2013) 4397–4403.
[82] G.K. Deshwal, S. Tiwari, A. Kumar, R.K. Raman, S. Kadyan, Review on factors affecting and control of post-acidification in yoghurt and related products, Trends Food Sci. Technol. (2021).
[83] L. Xu, S.-M. Yan, C.-B. Cai, Z.-J. Wang, X.-P. Yu, The feasibility of using near-infrared spectroscopy and chemometrics for untargeted detection of protein adulteration in yogurt: removing unwanted variations in pure yogurt, J. Anal. Methods Chem. (2013) 2013.
[84] O.G. Meza-Márquez, T. Gallardo-Velázquez, L. Dorantes-Álvarez, G. Osorio-Revilla, J.L. De La Rosa Arana, FT-MIR and Raman spectroscopy coupled to multivariate analysis for the detection of clenbuterol in murine model, Analyst 136 (2011) 3355–3365.
[85] R.M. El-Abassy, P. Donfack, A. Materny, Rapid determination of free fatty acid in extra virgin olive oil by Raman spectroscopy and multivariate analysis, J. Am. Oil Chem. Soc. 86 (2009) 507–511.
[86] B. Muik, B. Lendl, A. Molina-Dıaz, M.A.J. Ayora-Cañada, Direct, reagent-free determination of free fatty acid content in olive oil and olives by Fourier transform Raman spectrometry, Anal. Chim. Acta 487 (2003) 211–220.
[87] C. Choe, J. Schleusener, J. Lademann, M.E. Darvin, In vivo confocal Raman microscopic determination of depth profiles of the stratum corneum lipid organization influenced by application of various oils, J. Dermatol. Sci. 87 (2017) 183–191.
[88] Y. Song, C. Kim, J. Ahn, J. Woo, Y. Kim, H. Kim, Morphological and chemical structure of hydrothermally carbonized saccharides, Fibers Polym. 18 (2017) 1602–1608.
[89] K. Ilaslan, I.H. Boyaci, A. Topcu, Rapid analysis of glucose, fructose and sucrose contents of commercial soft drinks using Raman spectroscopy, Food Control. 48 (2015) 56–61.
[90] N.A. Karim, I.I., MuhamadDetection methods and advancement in analysis of food and beverages: a short review on adulteration and Halal authentication, in: Proceedings of the 3rd International Halal Conference (INHAC 2016), Springer, (2018) 397–414.
[91] B.R. Pinkard, D.J. Gorman, E.G. Rasmussen, V. Maheshwari, J.C. Kramlich, P.G. Reinhall, et al., Raman spectroscopic data from Formic Acid Decomposition in sub-critical and supercritical water, Data Brief. 29 (2020) 105312.
[92] Q. Wang, Z. Li, Z. Ma, L. Liang, Real time monitoring of multiple components in wine fermentation using an on-line auto-calibration Raman spectroscopy, Sens. Actuators B: Chem. 202 (2014) 426–432.
[93] C.A.T. Dos Santos, R.N. Páscoa, P.A. Porto, A.L. Cerdeira, J. González-Sáiz, C. Pizarro, et al., Raman spectroscopy for wine analyses: a comparison with near and mid infrared spectroscopy, Talanta 186 (2018) 306–314.

[94] T.-T. Pan, H. Pu, D.-W. Sun, Insights into the changes in chemical compositions of the cell wall of pear fruit infected by Alternaria alternata with confocal Raman microspectroscopy, Postharvest Biol. Technol. 132 (2017) 119–129.
[95] W.A. Tegegne, M.L. Mekonnen, A.B. Beyene, W.-N. Su, B.-J. Hwang, Sensitive and reliable detection of deoxynivalenol mycotoxin in pig feed by surface enhanced Raman spectroscopy on silver nanocubes@ polydopamine substrate, Spectrochim. Acta Part. A: Mol. Biomol. Spectrosc. 229 (2020) 117940.
[96] M. Petersen, Z. Yu, X. Lu, Application of Raman spectroscopic methods in food safety: a review, Biosensors 11 (2021) 187.
[97] O. Taylan, N. Cebi, M.T. Yilmaz, O. Sagdic, D. Ozdemir, M. Balubaid, Rapid detection of green-pea adulteration in pistachio nuts using Raman spectroscopy and chemometrics, J. Sci. Food Agric. 101 (2021) 1699–1708.
[98] M. Esteki, M. Cardador, N. Jurado-Campos, A. Martín-Gómez, L. Arce, J. Simal-Gandara, Innovations in analytical methods for food authenticity, Innovative Food Analysis, Elsevier, 2021.
[99] M. Gigli, S.M. Doglia, J.M. Millot, et al., Quantitative study of doxorubicin in living cell nuclei by microspectrofluorometry, Biochim. Biophys. Acta 950 (1988) 13e20.
[100] M. Gigli, W.D. Rasoanaivo, J.M. Millot, et al., Correlation between growth inhibition and intranuclear doxorubicin and 4'-deoxy-4'-iododoxorubicin quantitated in living K562 cells by microspectrofluorometry, Cancer Res. 49 (1989) 560e4.
[101] M. Gigli, S.M. Doglia, J.M. Millot, L. Valentini, M. Manfait, Quantitative study of doxorubicin in living cell nuclei by microspectrofluorometry, Biochimica Biophysica Acta (BBA)-Gene Struct. Expr. 950 (1988) 13–20.
[102] M. Gigli, T.W. Rasoanaivo, J.-M. Millot, P. Jeannesson, V. Rizzo, J.-C. Jardillier, et al., Correlation between growth inhibition and intranuclear doxorubicin and 4′-deoxy-4′-iododoxorubicin quantitated in living K562 cells by microspectrofluorometry, Cancer Res. 49 (1989) 560–564.
[103] C. Eliasson, P. Matousek, Noninvasive authentication of pharmaceutical products through packaging using partial offset Raman spectroscopy, Anal. Chem. 79 (2007) 1696e701.
[104] C. Eliasson, P. Matousek, Noninvasive authentication of pharmaceutical products through packaging using spatially offset Raman spectroscopy, Anal. Chem. 79 (2007) 1696–1701.
[105] M.C. Davies, J.S. Binns, C.D. Melia, et al., FT Raman spectroscopy of drugs in polymers, Int. J. Pharm. 66 (1990) 223e32.
[106] H. Huang, H. Shi, S. Feng, J. Lin, W. Chen, Y. Yu, et al., Quick detection of traditional Chinese medicine 'Atractylodis Macrocephalae Rhizoma'pieces by surface-enhanced Raman spectroscopy, Laser Phys. 23 (2012) 015601.
[107] R. Huang, R. Chen, Q. Chen, et al. Raman spectral study of anti-angiogenic drugs on the role of chick vascular, in: Q. Luo, L.V. Wang, V.V. Tuchin, et al., editors. Eighth International Conference on Photonics and Imaging in Biology and Medicine, Bellingham WA: SPIE (2009) 75191F.
[108] L. He, M. Lin, H. Li, et al., Surface-enhanced Raman spectroscopy coupled with dendritic silver nanosubstrate for detection of restricted antibiotics, J. Raman Spectrosc. 41 (2010) 739e44.
[109] L. He, M. Lin, H. Li, N.J. Kim, Surface-enhanced Raman spectroscopy coupled with dendritic silver nanosubstrate for detection of restricted antibiotics, J. Raman Spectrosc. 41 (2010) 739–744.
[110] G. Smulevich, J.M. Mauro, L.A. Fishel, A.M. English, J. Kraut, T.G. Spiro, Heme pocket interactions in cytochrome c peroxidase studied by site-directed mutagenesis and resonance Raman spectroscopy, Biochemistry 27 (1988) 5477–5485.

[111] R.A. Sulk, R.C. Corcoran, K.T. Carron, Surface-enhanced Raman scattering detection of amphetamine and methamphetamine by modification with 2- mercaptonicotinic acid, Appl. Spectrosc. 53 (1999) 954e9.
[112] K. Kneipp, A. Haka, H. Kneipp, et al., Surface-enhanced Raman spectroscopy in single living cells using gold nanoparticles, Appl. Spectrosc. 56 (2002) 150e4.
[113] K. Kneipp, A.S. Haka, H. Kneipp, K. Badizadegan, N. Yoshizawa, C. Boone, et al., Surface-enhanced Raman spectroscopy in single living cells using gold nanoparticles, Appl. Spectrosc. 56 (2002) 150–154.
[114] J. Kneipp, Nanosensors based on SERS for application living cells, in: K. Kneipp, M. Moskovits, H. Kneipp (Eds.), Surface Enhanced Raman Scattering: Physics and Applications, Springer-Verlag, Berlin Heidelberg, 2006.
[115] J. Kneipp, H. Kneipp, B. Wittig, K. Kneipp, Novel optical nanosensors for probing and imaging live cells, Nanomed. Nanotechnol. Biol. Med. 6 (2010) 214–226.
[116] K. Sokolov, P. Khodorchenko, A. Petukhov, I. Nabiev, G. Chumanov, T.M. Cotton, Contributions of short-range and classical electromagnetic mechanisms to surface-enhanced Raman scattering from several types of biomolecules adsorbed on cold-deposited island films, Appl. Spectrosc. 47 (1993) 515–522.
[117] C. Zavaleta, A. De La Zerda, Z. Liu, S. Keren, Z. Cheng, M. Schipper, et al., Noninvasive Raman spectroscopy in living mice for evaluation of tumor targeting with carbon nanotubes, Nano Lett. 8 (2008) 2800–2805.
[118] D. Zeisel, V. Deckert, R. Zenobi, T. Vo-Dinh, Near-field surface-enhanced Raman spectroscopy of dye molecules adsorbed on silver island films, Chem. Phys. Lett. 283 (1998) 381–385.
[119] V. Deckert, D. Zeisel, R. Zenobi, T. Vo-Dinh, Near-field surface-enhanced Raman imaging of dye-labeled DNA with 100-nm resolution, Anal. Chem. 70 (1998) 2646–2650.
[120] H. Huang, W. Chen, J. Pan, et al., SERS spectra of a single nasopharyngeal carcinoma cell based on intracellularly grown and passive uptake Au nanoparticles, Spectrosc 26 (2011) 187e94.
[121] J. Lin, R. Chen, S. Feng, et al., Rapid delivery of silver nanoparticles into living cells by electroporation for surface-enhanced Raman spectroscopy, Biosens. Bioelectron. 25 (2009) 388e94.
[122] J. Lin, R. Chen, S. Feng, Y. Li, Z. Huang, S. Xie, et al., Rapid delivery of silver nanoparticles into living cells by electroporation for surface-enhanced Raman spectroscopy, Biosens. Bioelectron. 25 (2009) 388–394.
[123] T.A. Jarvis, G.K. Bielmyer-Fraser, Accumulation and effects of metal mixtures in two seaweed species, Comp. Biochem. Physiol. Part. C: Toxicol. Pharmacol. 171 (2015) 28–33.
[124] C.T. Nguyen, J.T. Nguyen, S. Rutledge, et al., Detection of chronic lymphocytic leukemia cell surface markers using surface enhanced Raman scattering gold nanoparticles, Cancer Lett. 292 (2010) 91e7.
[125] C.T. Nguyen, J.T. Nguyen, S. Rutledge, J. Zhang, C. Wang, G.C. Walker, Detection of chronic lymphocytic leukemia cell surface markers using surface enhanced Raman scattering gold nanoparticles, Cancer Lett. 292 (2010) 91–97.
[126] D.T. Nguyen, D.-J. Kim, K.-S. Kim, Controlled synthesis and biomolecular probe application of gold nanoparticles, Micron 42 (2011) 207–227.
[127] H. Zhou, D. Yang, N.P. Ivleva, N.E. Mircescu, R. Niessner, C. Haisch, SERS detection of bacteria in water by in situ coating with Ag nanoparticles, Anal. Chem. 86 (2014) 1525–1533.
[128] E. Witkowska, T. Szymborski, A. Kamińska, J. Waluk, Polymer mat prepared via Forcespinning™ as a SERS platform for immobilization and detection of bacteria from blood plasma, Mater. Sci. Eng. C. 71 (2017) 345–350.

[129] Z. Guo, M. Wang, A.O. Barimah, Q. Chen, H. Li, J. Shi, et al., Label-free surface enhanced Raman scattering spectroscopy for discrimination and detection of dominant apple spoilage fungus, Int. J. Food Microbiol. 338 (2021) 108990.
[130] R. Panneerselvam, G.-K. Liu, Y.-H. Wang, J.-Y. Liu, S.-Y. Ding, J.-F. Li, et al., Surface-enhanced Raman spectroscopy: bottlenecks and future directions, Chem. Commun. 54 (2018) 10–25.
[131] M.J. Pelletier, Quantitative analysis using Raman spectrometry, Appl. Spectrosc. 57 (2003) 20A–42A.
[132] A.-K. Kniggendorf, C. Wetzel, B. Roth, Microplastics detection in streaming tap water with Raman spectroscopy, Sensors 19 (2019) 1839.
[133] L. Zada, H.A. Leslie, A.D. Vethaak, G.H. Tinnevelt, J.J. Jansen, J.F. De Boer, et al., Fast microplastics identification with stimulated Raman scattering microscopy, J. Raman Spectrosc. 49 (2018) 1136–1144.
[134] L. Lv, L. He, S. Jiang, J. Chen, C. Zhou, J. Qu, et al., In situ surface-enhanced Raman spectroscopy for detecting microplastics and nanoplastics in aquatic environments, Sci. Total. Environ. 728 (2020) 138449.

CHAPTER FIVE

Chromatographic methods for the analysis of oils and fats

Gunawan Indrayanto[1] and Abdul Rohman[2]
[1]Faculty of Pharmacy, Surabaya University, Surabaya, Indonesia
[2]Faculty of Pharmacy, Gadjah Mada University, Jogyakarta, Indonesia

5.1 Introduction

According to the United States Patent and Trademark Office [1], "oil" can be defined as a substance that is in a viscous liquid state ("oily") at ambient temperatures or slightly warmer and is both hydrophobic (immiscible with water) and lipophilic (miscible with other oils, literally). The term "oil" is used to describe of any substance that does not mix with water and has a greasy feel, such as petroleum (or crude oil) and heating oil, regardless of its chemical structure. Edible oil is fat of plant, animal, or microbial origin, which is liquid at room temperature and can be used as food; examples of edible vegetable oils include olive oil, palm oil, soybean oil, canola oil, pumpkin seed oil, corn oil, sunflower oil, safflower oil, peanut oil, grape seed oil, sesame oil, argan oil, and rice bran oil. Fish oil is an example of edible oil of animal origin.

In general, fats consist of a wide range of compounds that are generally soluble in organic solvents but insoluble in water. Fats are generally triacylglycerols (TAG), tri-esters of glycerol and fatty acids. Fats may be either solid or liquid at normal room temperature, depending on their structure and composition. The terms "oils," "fats," and "lipids" are all used to refer to fats; Oil refers to fats that are liquid at normal room temperature, while fat is usually used to refer to lipids that are solid at normal room temperature. Lipid is used to refer to both liquid and solid fats, along with other related substances [1]. Vegetable oils are generally named as "fixed oils" in United States Pharmacopoeia-National Formulary (USP-NF); the term fixed oils differentiate them from the essential oils and volatile petrochemical oils.

Food Quality Analysis.
DOI: https://doi.org/10.1016/B978-0-323-95988-9.00004-7

Fixed oils are obtained by expression or extraction; their consistency depends to the temperature, some are liquid (oils), others are semisolid (fats), and solid (tallows) at ambient temperature [2]. Hydrogenated vegetable oil is a mixture of triglycerides of fatty acids; their melting range, iodine value, and saponification value differ depending on the type (I or II) [3]

5.2 Quality assessment of oils and fats

In 1992, International Union of Pure and Applied Chemistry, Commission on Oils, Fats and Derivatives (IUPAC) [4] published standard methods for the analysis of oils, fats, and derivate. General chapter of the USP45-NF40 <401> [5] describes various general tests to determine the quality fats and oils as follows: specific gravity, melting temperature, acid value, ester value, hydroxyl value, iodine value, peroxide value, saponification value, unsaponifiable value, solidification temperature of fatty acids, fatty acid compositions, omega-3 fatty acid determination and profile, water and sedimentation in fixed oils, anisidine value, total oxidation value, trace metals, and sterol compositions. The World Health Organization [6] describes detailed protocol measuring fatty acid profile of foods, with emphasis on monitoring trans-fatty acids originating from partially hydrogenated oils; sampling plan, sample collection and storage, and analytical methodology were described and discussed. Food Safety and Standards Authority of India (FSSAI) [7] describes general test for fats and oils, identification test for several oils, and method of determination of certain compounds in oil. A review on the analytical methods for evaluating the quality of edible oils and fats using the standard method of Japanese Oil Chemists' Society has been published by Endo [8]; the author stated that the application of nondestructive methods such as infrared, near-infrared, terahertz spectrophotometry proton nuclear magnetic resonance and ^{13}C nuclear magnetic resonance are expected to be applied in the near future. News Medical Life Sciences [9] summarized seven important parameters for analysis of edible oils and fats that have been described by several official guidelines, for example, Association of Official Analytical Chemist (AOAC), American Society of Testing Materials (ASTM), United States Pharmacopoeia (USP),

American Oil Chemists' Society (AOCS), etc.; all methods of analysis were described in brief. The AOCS [10] has described various methods of analysis of lipids, that is, method of solid-phase extractions, preparation of derivatives of fatty acids for chromatographic analysis, fatty acid analysis, identification of fatty acid methyl esters (FAME) using mass spectrometry and other chromatographic methods; the readers can select each of the methods directly from the described URL. Some of testing methods that are described by International Olive Council (IOC) for olive oils, for example, determination of fatty acid ester by gas chromatography (COI/T.20/Doc. No 33), determination of sterols composition (COI/T.20/Doc. N° 26), determination of stigmastadienes in vegetable oils (COI/T-20/Doc. N°11), determination of peroxide value (COI/T.20/Doc. No 35), etc. can be applied for quality check of other vegetables oils [11]. The International Organization for Standardization published paid methods for the quality assessment of fats and oils; the methods can be obtained via this URL [12].

The quality assessment of fats and oils entails a nonspecific method of analysis, for example, specific gravity, melting temperature, acid value, ester value, hydroxyl value, iodine value etc., and a specific method of analysis, for example, identification methods, fatty acid profiles, sterols compositions, etc., that are usually performed using chromatographic methods of analysis. Thin-layer chromatography (TLC), gas chromatography with flame ionization detection (GC-FID), and high-performance liquid chromatography (HPLC; refractive index detector [RID], fluorescence detector, ultraviolet–visible [UV–VIS] detector) were applied by for the quality assessment of oil and fats as described by Apte [2], IUPAC [4], WHO [6], FSSAI [7], and Endo [8], but general chapter of USP45-NF39 <401> [5] describes only GC method, while identification of fixed oils using TLC was described by the general chapter of USP44-NF39 <202> [13]. Application of nondestructive spectroscopic methods of analysis has also been recommended [8]. Taher et al. [14] published a detailed review article on the application of chemometrics for tracing the origin of oils that appeared between 2013 to 2020. European Pharmacopeia (EP) 10 [15] (Section 2.3.2) described identification method of fatty oils using TLC; GC-FID was described in Section 2.4.22 and Section 2.4.23.

Detailed discussion on the chromatographic methods of analysis of fats and oils and their method validations will be presented in the following sections.

5.3 Chromatographic based techniques

5.3.1 Application of TLC for quality control of edible fats and oils

5.3.1.1 Qualitative analysis

For quality control (QC) purposes, TLC methods can be applied for qualitative (identification) and quantitative analysis. Official method of qualitative identification of fixed- and fatty-oils have been described by the USP [13] and EP 10 in Section 2.3.2 [15]. These methods are summarized in Table 5.1. System suitability test (SST) requirements for identification of fixed oils are described by the USP [13]; The R_F values for the four principal spots for USP Corn Oil RS are 0.39, 0.45, 0.51, and 0.56, and the values for the two principal spots for USP Olive Oil RS are 0.39 and 0.45. The requirement of SST was not available in EP, but typical TLC chromatograms of 16 oils were presented for both methods A and B [15]. Evaluation of the TLC method is performed by visual observation; R_F of principle spots of sample solution should correspond to the standard solution.

The manual techniques of TLC methods of identification (Table 5.1) have shown poor reproducibility due to the strong influence of experimental conditions [16]. To have more reliable results for the manual identification of botanicals (including oils) using the profile of TLC images, a completed and comprehensive method validation should be performed as described in the previous publications [17,18]. Ofori et al. [19] reported high-performance TLC (HPTLC) fingerprinting of some sandalwood essential oils and compared the R_F values, color, and intensities of the spots/peaks of the samples. Srivastava et al. [20] reported a method validation for the assessment of TLC fingerprinting using HPTLC densitogram, using similarity evaluation (SA) by calculating the correlation coefficient, congruence coefficient, and similarity index of samples and standards. Detailed discussion regarding the evaluation using SA can be referred to a previous study [21]. Evaluation of TLC chromatograms using SA was already described in the Chinese Pharmacopoeia 2015 [22]. HPTLC profiles of some different Egyptian Olive varieties could also be directly generated using Image software after auto processing and enhancing the TLC images by XnView 2.40 freeware, then evaluated by chemometrics methods [23]. The application of SA and chemometrics methods for the

Table 5.1 Official identification of fixed and fatty oils using TLC.

Method [Reference]	Stationary phase	Mobile phase	Standard solution	Analysis	Detection
Method I [13]	HPTLC plate: (20 cm × 10 cm, silica gel 60 RP-18, 0.15–0.2 mm layer, 4–8 μm particle size)	MP1: ethyl ether; MP2: methylene chloride, glacial acetic acid, and acetone (20:40:50)	Appropriate USP RS (20 mg or 1 drop/3 mL methylene chloride	Develop two times over a path of 0.5 cm using MP1, after drying develop two times over 8 cm using MP2	100 mg/mL of phosphomolybdic acid in 96% alcohol (120°C, 1 min); examine in daylight
Method II [13]	HPTLC plate: (20 cm × 10 cm, silica gel 60 RP-18, 0.15–0.2 mm layer, 4–8 μm particle size	Methylene chloride, glacial acetic acid, and acetone (20:40:50)	25 μL of the appropriate USP RS/ 3 mL of methylene chloride	Predevelop the plate with methylene chloride to the upper edge. Dry (120°C, 10 min); Develop over a path of 7 cm	100 mg/mL of phosphomolybdic acid in 96% alcohol (120°C, 1 min); examine in daylight
A [15]	HPTLC plate: RP-18	MP1: ethyl ether; MP2: methylene chloride, glacial acetic acid, and acetone (20:40:50)	Maize oil R (20 mg/1 drop in 3 mL methylene chloride)	Develop two times over a path of 0.5 cm using MP1, after drying develop two times over 8 cm using MP2	100 mg/mL of phosphomolybdic acid in 96% alcohol (120°C, 3 min); examine in daylight
B [15]	HPTLC plate: RP-18	Methylene chloride, glacial acetic acid, and acetone (20:40:50)	Maize oil R (20 mg/1 drop in 3 mL methylene chloride	Develop over a path of 7 cm	100 mg/mL of phosphomolybdic acid in 96% alcohol (120°C, 3 min; examine in daylight

evaluation of the TLC chromatograms are recommended by the authors, instead of using visual comparison [13,15] (Table 5.1) and Ref. [19], due to the less accuracy and preciseness of the manual method; both methods of SA and chemometrics and their validation method of analysis should be described in the next edition of the pharmacopoeias.

5.3.1.2 Quantitative analysis

For quantitative analysis of certain compounds in fats and oils, the method used should be first verified or validated prior to routine applications. It is recommended to refer the official method validation of the current USP-NF, that is, general chapter <1225> [24], <1226> [25], <1210> [26], and <1010> [27]. The validation parameters that should be validated include specificity, linearity, accuracy, precision (repeatability, intermediate precision), range, detection limit, quantification limit, and robustness. Ferenczi-Fodor et al. [28] described and discussed the important validation parameters that should be evaluated for quantitative analysis using TLC methods. The target of the TLC densitometric chromatogram should be evaluated for its identity and purity; identical R_F does not mean identical compounds, and one peak does not mean a single compound. Detailed discussions on the chromatographic method of analysis for herbal drugs are given in our previous chapter [29]. Examples of TLC quantitative analysis of certain compounds commonly occurring in fats and oils that appeared in the Journal of Planar Chromatography-Modern TLC (Springer) are summarized in Table 5.2.

The fifth column of Table 5.2 shows that all the publications were not fully validated according the current USP-NF as described above. Methods of evaluating the repeatability and intermediate precision of all publications listed in Table 5.2 are not correct. Such evaluation should be performed by completed analysis methods instead of using standard solutions only. Only Refs. [33,34] reported selectivity by evaluating the identity and purity of the target peaks in samples; without this evaluation, the identity and purity of the target peak is samples cannot be confirmed, so that the results of quantitative analyses might not be accurate.

5.3.2 GC-FID and GC-MS for quality assessment of fats and oils

5.3.2.1 General principle

GC equipped with a nonspecific detector FID is used as the common official method of quality assessment (Section 5.3.2.2). Therefore in

Table 5.2 Quantitative analysis of certain common compounds in fats and oils and other products using thin-layer chromatography (TLC).

Sample	Compound	Plate (mobile phase)	Detection	Validation	Ref.
Vegetables oils	α-γ and δ Tocopherol	HPTLC silica gel 60 (chloroform)	Bipyridyl in MeOH (0.5%): $FeCl_3$ in MeOH (0.2%) (1;1); densitometric: Cano Scan Lide20, 600 × 1200 dpi	Linearity and other validation parameters were not reported	[30]
Fish oil	Vitamin D3	HPTLC silica gel 60 F254 (chloroform–ether 9:1 (v/v)	UV–Vis 280 nm	Linearity, limit of determination (LOD), limit of quantification (LOQ), repeatability, and intermediate precision (analysis of standard solutions), accuracy by standard addition, selectivity was missing	[31]
Sunflower oil	β-carotene	HPTLC silica gel 60 (petroleum ether–hexane–acetone 2:1:1 (v/v)	UV–Vis 450 nm	Instrument precision, linearity, LOD, LOQ, repeatability (analysis carotene band 7 × , selectivity (R_F, spectra, purity was missing), accuracy was not reported	[32]

(Continued)

Table 5.2 (Continued)

Sample	Compound	Plate (mobile phase)	Detection	Validation	Ref.
Palmarosa oil	Geraniol	HPTLC silica gel 60 F_{254} (toluene–ethyl acetate (92.5:7.5, v/v)	UV–Vis 400 nm (vanillin–H_2SO_4)	Selectivity (identity and purity), linearity, repeatability (analyzing six bands of standards), LOD, LOQ, accuracy method was not reported)	[33]
Dietary supple ments	Omega-3 fatty acids	Various plates of silica gel 60 F254, RP 18F, Cellulose F_{254} (toluene–n-propanol–glacial acetic acid (20:2:0.1, v/v)	After samples were prepared[a], densitometry was performed at UV–Vis 580 nm	Selectivity (identity and purity), linearity, LOD, LOQ, repeatability, and intermediate precision (analysis of standard solutions), accuracy by standard addition	[34]

[a]Methods are elaborated in the original publication.

addition of the SST test already described in [5], and EP 10 discussed in Section 2.4.22 [15], it is recommended to confirm the identity and the purity of the target peaks using method that described by the Eurachem Guide [35]. Retention time (Rt) or relative retention time (RRt) of the target peaks measured using at least three different GC conditions should be identical to the standards. If the chromatography instrument is coupled with mass spectrometry (Ms) detector, for confirmation of the identity of the target peaks in samples, the readers should consult the guidance of the Food and Drug Administration (FDA), Office of Regulatory Affairs [36], and Commission Implementing Regulation (EU) [37].

According to the current USP-online, the official method of identification of oils using GC entails the determination of the compound profile/composition as described in Section 5.3.2.2. Other methods of identification involve comparing the chromatographic similarity between sample and oil reference standard and/or determination of the minimum content of a certain secondary metabolite as described in the monograph of anise oil [38]; if their concentrations do not meet the requirements, the presence of the metabolites should be confirmed using electron impact (EI)- and chemical ionization- gas chromatography-mass spectrometry (CI-GC-MS); the m/z of molecular- and one fragment-ion of foeniculin and myristicin should be observed. Unfortunately, the described requirements do not meet the acceptance criteria of the FDA, Office of Regulatory Affairs [36] and Commission Implementing Regulation (EU) [37] According to these official guidance's, it needs at least 2 ions with accuracy <5 ppm [36] or one molecular ion and one fragment ion with ion ratio within $\pm 40\%$ of the standard [37]. The authors recommend USP to revise the monograph of anise oil [38] by completing the requirements as described in the guidelines of the FDA and EU. Prior to the application of any method of the pharmacopoeias for routine applications, it must be first verified or validated as described in Section 5.3.1.2.

5.3.2.2 General official methods

The general methods of quality assessment of fats and oils using GC will be briefly described in the following sections. Detailed methods can be referred to in the guidelines.

5.3.2.2.1 Fatty acid composition

5.3.2.2.1.1 USP-NF <401> Methods [5]: GC equipped with FID (260°C), a splitless injection system, and a 0.53-mm × 30-m fused-silica capillary column bonded with a 1.0-μm layer of phase G16 (70°C, 2 min, then 5°C/min to 240°C for 5 min), injection port temperature at 220°C, carrier gas He (50 cm/s), standard solutions Nu-Chek 17A and Nu-Chek 19A (Nu-Chek-Prep, Inc., Elysian, MN 56028). SST of the method: RRts are 0.87 (methyl palmitate), 0.99 (methyl stearate), 1.0 (methyl oleate); the resolution (Rs) between methyl stearate and methyl oleate is NLT 1.5; and relative standard deviation (RSD) of the peak area responses for the palmitate and stearate peaks for replicate injections is NMT 6.0%, and RSD of their ratio of peak is NMT 1.0%. Percent composition can be calculated as (individual peak response/total peaks responses) × 100. The composition of fatty acid profile is described in each of the monograph.

5.3.2.2.1.2 EP 10 In EP 10 Section 2.4.22 [15], only the GC conditions were described. SST depends on the mixture of reference standards used; detail of the method, including samples preparations, can be referred to this section.

Method A:

This method is not applicable for oils containing glycerides of fatty acids with an epoxy-, hydro epoxy-, hydro peroxy-, cyclopropyl, or cyclopropenyl-group or those that contain a large proportion of fatty acids of chain length less than eight carbon atoms or to oils with an acid value > 2.0.

GC-FID (250°C), and a 10–30 m fused silica, glass, or quartz (0.2–0.8 mm) macrogol 20,000R, film thickness 0.1–0.5 μm (isothermal 200°C for 30 m column, or 170°C–230°C, 3°C/min), split ratio 1:1000 or less, carrier gas (He or H_2 1.3 mL/min), injection port 250°C,

Method B:

This method is not applicable for oils containing glycerides of fatty acids with an epoxy-, hydro epoxy-, hydro peroxy-, cyclopropyl, or cyclopropenyl-group or to oils with an acid value > 2.0.

GC-FID (250°C), and a 30 m fused silica, glass, or quartz (0.25 mm) macrogol 20,000R, film thickness 0.5 μm (100°C: 0–15 min, 100°C–225°C: 15–36 min, then 225°C: 36–61 min), split ratio 1:100 or less, carrier gas (He or H_2 0.9 mL/min), injection port 250°C.

Method C:

This method is not applicable for oils containing glycerides of fatty acids with an epoxy-, hydro epoxy-, hydro peroxy-, cyclopropyl, or cyclopropenyl-group, and conjugated polyunsaturated and acetylenic compounds because of partial or completed destruction of these groups.

5.3.2.2.2 Sterols composition

5.3.2.2.2.1 USP-NF The official method of determining sterols composition according to the general chapter of the current USP-NF <401> [5] is by using GC equipped with FID (290°C), a split ratio 1: 50 or 1: 100, a glass or fused-silica capillary column 20–30 m in length, internal diameter 0.25–0.32 mm, entirely coated with a 0.10- to 0.30-μm layer of stationary phase G27 or G36 (260°C ± 5°C), injection port temperature at 280°C, carrier gas He (25–50 cm/s, or H_2 30–50 cm/s); SST using reference solution; Rt of the peak of β-sitosterol should be 20 ± 5 min, and the principle peaks of sterols should be separated (cholesterol, brassicasterol, campesterol, and ß-sitosterol [Reference E] or campesterol, stigmasterol, β-sitosterol, and Δ7-stigmastenol [Reference F]). Relative retention times of the sterols in standard solutions for two stationary phases G27 and G7 are listed in Table 12 of the chapter USP-NF that described by Ref. [5]; details of the methods of preparation of standard (E and F) and test solutions have been described. The readers can refer to this chapter of the USP-NF [5].

5.3.2.2.2.2 EP 10 The official method of determination according to EP 10 Section 2.4.23 [15] is by using GC equipped with FID (2900°C), a split ratio 1:50 (H_2) or 1:100 (He) is used, a fused-silica capillary column 20–30 m in length, internal diameter 0.25–0.32 mm, stationary phase: phenyl(5)methyl(95) poly siloxane R or cyanopropyl(7)methyl(860 poly siloxane (0.25 μm, 260°C), injection port temperature at 280°C, carrier gas He (25–35 cm/s, or H_2 30–50 cm/s). SST: four peaks of cholesterol, brassicasterol, campesterol, and ß-sitosterol (reference solution a), or campesterol, stigmasterol, β-sitosterol, and Δ7-stigmastenol (Reference b). Details of the methods of preparation of standard (a and b) and test solutions have been described. The readers can refer to this chapter of the EP 10.

5.3.2.2.3 Omega-3 fatty acid determination and profiles

The procedures used to determine eicosapentaenoic acid (EPA: C20:5 *n*-3), docosahexaenoic acid (DHA) (C22:6 *n*-3), and total omega-3 either as triglycerides or as ethyl esters are described by the USP [5]. Instrument: GC equipped with FID (270°C) and a 0.53-mm × 30-m fused-silica capillary column bonded with a 0. 20 μm layer of phase G16 (split injection: 170°C, 2 min, 3°C/min to 240°C, 2.5 min; splitless injection: 90°C, 30°C/min to 170°C then 3°C/min to 240°C, 2 min), injection port: split: 250°C, splitless: 9°C–250°C, carrier gas He (1 mL/min). Detailed SST and method of determination of EPA, DHA, and omega-3 can be referred to this general chapter the USP-NF [5]. Method of determination of EPA, DHA, and total omega-3 are also described by to EP 10 Section 2.4.29 [15].

5.3.2.3 Application of gas chromatographic methods for quality assessment of fats and oils

Waktola et al. [39] published a review article on the application of advanced one- and multidimensional GC-MS for the analysis of fatty acids and TAG. Mota et al. [40] recently published a detailed review article on the quality assessment of seed and vegetables oils using one-dimensional GC-MS and multidimensional gas chromatography (GC × GC-MS) methodologies. Determination of fatty acids, FAME, triacyl glycerol, volatile organic compounds, phytosterol etc., and methods of authentication of vegetables oils were summarized and discussed by the researchers. Precise and informative application notes for analysis of fatty acids, triglycerides, sterols, and essential oils using GC-FID and GC-MS were issued by Phenomenex [41]. Application notes for comprehensive analysis of fatty acids, FAME, and triglycerides using GC are published by Agilent [42]. Some examples of publications on the specific quality assessment of fats and oils are summarized in Table 5.3.

As shown in the sixth column of Table 5.3, validation method of analysis was not completed reported as required (see Section 5.3.1.2). The most important validation parameter in any chromatographic methods is the selectivity, that is, the identity and purity of all target peaks in samples, and this should be evaluated and confirmed as described in Section 5.3.1.2 and Section 3.2.1. For further discussions regarding the importance of the method validation by using chromatography, the readers can refer to our previous review articles [29] and [52].

5.3.3 LC and related techniques for analysis of fats and oils

5.3.3.1 Standard methods for quality assessment

Standard methods for the quality assessment of fats and oils using HPLC have been published by IUPAC [4], that is, (1) determination of triglycerides in vegetable oils (HPLC-RID), (2) tocopherols and tocotrienols in vegetable oils and fats (HPLC-fluorescence detector: excitation 290 nm, emission 330 nm), (3) polymerized triglycerides in oils and fats (HPLC-RID), (4) benzo(α)pyrene in edible oils and fats

Table 5.3 Application of gas chromatographic methods for quality assessment of fats and oils.

Samples	Issues	Sample preparation	GC conditions	Results	Validation	Ref.
Vegetable oils and corn oils	Analysis of trans-fat in edible oils with cooking process	Derivatization of fatty acid methyl esters was performed by BF_3/MeOH (AOAC 969.33)	GC-FID (285°C); column: SP-2560 (100 m × 0.25 mm, 0.20 μm film), 100°C, 4 min to 225°C, 3°C/min, 20 min; split ratio: 1:200, injector 225°C, He 0.75 mL/min,	GC-FID can be applied for analyzing trans-fat in edible oils.	Not reported	[43]
27 Vegetable oil (Vo) samples GC-MSD	Determination of botanical origin of Vo	Sample dissolved in CH_2Cl_2, derivatized using TMSH	GC-MSD (70 eV); column: DB-5 Ms (30 m × 0.25 mm × 25 μm), 50°C–130°C, 30°C/min, 130°C–300°C, 10°C/min	Cluster analysis using nine dominant fatty acids can differentiate samples with different botanical origin	Not reported	[44]
Cocoa butter, palm oil, canola oil	Determination of tri acetyl glycerol	Sample and internal standard were dissolved in CH_2Cl_2	GC-FID (350°C); column: ultra-alloy (30 × 0.25 mm, 0.10 μm), 250°C to 360°C, 4°C/min; injector 350°C	TAG compositions in samples were in good agreement with literature.	LOD and LOQ were reported; selectivity, accuracy, and precision were not reported	[45]

(Continued)

Table 5.3 (Continued)

Samples	Issues	Sample preparation	GC conditions	Results	Validation	Ref.
Commercial vegetables, animals' oils, and fats produced in Romania and Malaysia	Validation method for deter mination of fatty acid profile in food	Samples were prepared according to ISO 661, 17189, 12966-2	GC-MS; column: TR-FAME (60 m × 0.25 mm, 0.25 μm) of 70% cyanopropyl and 30% polysilphenyl-siloxane, 100°C, 0. 2 min, to 240°C, 2°C/min, 15 min; ion source 250°C, SIM	The proposed method could be considered an effective tool for analyzing the fatty acid profile of food	Linearity, working range, sensitivity, repea tability, inter mediate precision, accuracy, and robustness were reported; selectivity was not reported	[46]
Commercial camelia oils (Co)	Detection of adulteration by using fingerprints of fatty acids (GC-FID), and phytosterols (GC-Ms)	Co was diluted with hexane and mixed with KOH-MeOH; Co + IS was then saponified with MeOH-KOH	GC-FID, column: CP-Sil 88 (0.25 μm, 60 m × 0.25 mm, 60°C, 3 min to 175°C, 5°C/min, 15 min then to 220°C, 2°C/min. 10 min. GC-EIMS, column: DB-5 Ms (0.25 mm, 30 m × 0.25 mm), 200°C, 1 min, to 300°C, 10°C/min, 18 min, ion source 290°C, EI: *m/z* 50 to 500	Co can be differentiated using partial least squares discriminant analysis (PLS-DA), 22 key markers can be identified; PLS can be applied to determination of the adulterants in Co	PCA was not validated, PLS-DA was validated using sevenfold cross validation, PLS was validated using R^2, RMSE, RMSECV, RMSEP, the identities of squalene, sterols, and triterpenes were not confirmed	[47]

Flaxseed oils (Fo) were obtained from 40 samples of flaxseed (Qinghai, China)	Determination of flaxseed oil adulteration based on fatty acid profiles and chemo metrics	KOH 1 M was added to Fo + IS, refluxed, cool, and added n-heptane for FAME extraction	GC-FID (250°C), column: Wonda Cap WAX (60 m × 0.25 mm, 0.25 μm), 100°C, 13 min, to 180°C, 10°C/min, 6 min, then to 200°C, 1°C/min, and to 230°C, 4°C/min, 10 min; injector 250°C	DA methods could identify oil adulterants in Fo (<20%). SA (heat map), if the concentrations of adulterants were 10%–50%.	PCA: no validation was reported; CDA: leave-one-out cross-validation; SA: no validation was reported	[48]
Extra virgin olive oil (EVO)	Determination of 3-and 2-monochloro propanediol (MCPD) esters and glycidol esters in edible oils	Methods of AOCS No. Cd 29b-13 and Cd 29c-13	GC-MS/MS, column: DB-17-Ms (30m × 0.25 mm, 0.25 μm), He (1.2 mL/min), multiple reaction monitoring (MRM)	The proposed automated procedures can be applied to determine MCPD and glycidol ester in EVO	Linearity, LOD, LOQ, precision, and accuracy were reported; confir mation of peak identity using Ms/MS was missing	[49]
Commercial olive oil, corn oil, soybean oil and canola oil	analysis of pesticides in edible oils	Sample extraction, lipid/matrix cleanup, and water removal/ drying (for details, please refer to the original publication	GC-MS/MS; column: two fused silica HP-5Ms UI (15 m × 0.25 mm, 0.25 μm) connected by a purged ultimate union, 60°C, 1 min; to 170°C, 40°C/min, 310°C, 10°C/ min, 3 min, EI (280°C), MRM	Recovery of 95% of tested pesticides >70%, RSD reproducibility (< 15%) in all sample	Accuracy, precision, and LOQ were reported in olive, soybean, corn, and canola oils; confir mation of peak identity using Ms/MS was missing	[50]

(Continued)

Table 5.3 (Continued)

Samples	Issues	Sample preparation	GC conditions	Results	Validation	Ref.
Virgin coconut oil (VCO) from different brands	Determination of fatty acid in raw, cooking VCO and food preparations	Oil, prepared food + KOH-MeOH (0.5 M), vortexed 2 min, 2 min, + n-hexane, vortexed, 2 min	GC-FID (255°C), column: DB-5Ms (30 m × 250 μm, 0.25 μm), 80°C to 170°C, 10°C/min then to 230°C, 3°C/min, 24 min. Injection port 250°C	The profile of the fatty acids in coconut oil is modified by the addition of other ingredients; heating the pure oils does not change the fatty acid profile	Linearity was reported, but other validation parameters were missing. Selectivity was reported by comparing Rt only.	[51]

AOCS, American Oil Chemists' Society; *DA*, discriminant analysis; *EIMS*, electron impact mass spectrometry; *GC-FID*, gas chromatography with flame ionization detection; *ISO*, International Organization for Standardization; *RMSE*, root mean square error; *RMSECV*, root mean square error of cross validation; *RMSEP*, root mean square of prediction; *SIM*, selected ion monitoring; *TAG*, triacylglycerols. *TMSH*, trimethylsulfonium hydroxide.

(HPLC-fluorescence detector: excitation 384 nm, emission 406 nm), and (5) phospholipid profile of lecithin (HPLC-UV 206 nm). The detailed methods can be referred to in this standard book [4]. Some other standard methods using LC have been described by AOCS, for example, the analysis of used frying oils and fats using size-exclusion chromatography [53], trans poly unsaturated fatty acids using HPLC and GC [54], and determination of oxidized monomeric, dimeric, and oligomeric TAG, as well as diacylglycerols and free fatty acids using combination of solid phase extraction and high-pressure size-exclusion chromatography [55].

The most noteworthy advantage of HPLC/LC compared to GC methods is preventing the possible degradations of some unsaturated TAG at high temperature [56].

5.3.3.2 Application of liquid chromatographic methods for quality assessment of fats and oils

Some applications of LC/HPLC for the quality control or quality assessment of fats and oils are summarized in Table 5.4. As discussed above in the section of TLC and GC, not all publications reported complete validation of the proposed methods. Without any validation data, the reliability of the conclusions of the methods cannot be confirmed, and they may not be replicated by other researchers.

5.4 Conclusions, recommendations, and future trends

As discussed above, for carrying out quality assessment of (edible) fats and oils according to the official guidelines is not simple and cheap; it needs suitable equipment, references standards, extractions, measurements including SST's evaluation of method, and verification/validation. Some nonspecific and specific evaluations that are described in of the monograph of oil/fat should be performed. Specific tests consisted of qualitative identification and quantitative determination of certain or group of compounds. The possible contaminants of certain metals such as arsenic, cadmium, copper, iron, mercury, lead, nickel, and zinc should be evaluated [5]. General methods for the determination of the metals using atomic absorption spectroscopy (AAS) is described by general chapter of

Table 5.4 Application of liquid chromatographic methods for quality assessment of fats and oils.

Samples	Issues	Sample preparation	LC conditions	Results	Validation	Ref.
Edible vegetable oils	Analysis of FAME in oxidized oils using HPLC-UV-evaporative light scattering detector (ELSD; detectors in series)	Derivatization using NaOMe; FAME was dissolved in hexane	HPLC-UV-ELSD: LiChrospher, Si 60, 250 mm × 4 mm, 5 μm): n-heptane/diethyl ether (82:18, v/v), 1 mL/min; UV 234 and 268 nm; ELSD (nebulizer: 35°C, tube 40°C, 25 psi gas flow)	ELSD showed higher hydroperoxide concentrations after the total depletion of tocopherols; linoleate was the predominant oxidation product; hydroperoxide compounds were degradation products of oils containing linolenic acid	No validation data were reported	[57]

Commercial edible oils; adulterated oils were self-prepared	Quantification of TAG using offline 2D-LC-APCI–MS	Oil samples dissolved in hexane, then mixture diluted with isopropanol	Optimization for separation of TAG was performed by reversed phase (RP)-HPLC; 1D-, 2D-LC using Zorbax Eclipse + phenyl-hexyl (4.6 × 250 mm, 5 μm), APCI-MS; for method details, see original publication	40 TAG (soybean oils), 50 TAG (peanut oils), 44 (lord oils) can be identified and quantified; PCA analysis can be used for the identification of different plant oils; 5% adulterations using lord oils can be identified by PCA	No detailed validation methods were reported; precision and accuracy of the off-line 2D-phenyl-hexyl–HPLC–Ms method was compared with standard GC-FID methods	[56]
Edible oils	Direct quantitative determination of major oxidation products in edible oils using normal phase HPLC-DAD	Oil samples were dissolved in heptane; derivatization: using NaOMe; FAME was dissolved in hexane (for comparison)	HPLC-DAD: LiChrospher, Si 60, 250 mm × 4 mm, 5 μm): n-heptane: diethyl ether (82:18, v/v), 1 mL/min. UV: 234 and 268 nm	The method can be applied for analyzing mono-hydroperoxy-dienes in edible oils without applying any isolation or derivatization step; results of direct analysis similar to FAME analysis	Linearity, LOD, LOQ, accuracy, and precision were reported; selectivity was not reported	[58]

(Continued)

Table 5.4 (Continued)

Samples	Issues	Sample preparation	LC conditions	Results	Validation	Ref.
Edible vegetable oils	Analyzing saturated fatty aldehydes, using a turn-on fluorescent probe	Oil samples dissolved in ACN, then derivatized using fluorescence reagents	HPLC-Fluorescence detector; C18 column (150 × 4.6 mm, 5 μm), MeOH-H_2O (80: 20, v/v), 1.0 mL/min; excitation 415, emission 462 nm	The fluorescent probe has been successfully used for the qualitative and quantitative detection of fatty aldehydes in edible vegetable oil samples	Data of linearity, LOD, LOQ, and accuracy were reported, but the methods were missing. Selectivity was not reported in detail	[59]
Sixteen different types of commercial olive oils, that is, extra virgin olive oils, ecological extra virgin olive oils, and refined olive oils	Analyzing polycyclic aromatic hydrocarbons (PAH) in commercial olive oils using HPLC/GC/MS	Samples were prepared using SPE, detailed method and its schematic of HPLC/GC/Ms system can be referred to in the original publication	HPLC/GC/MS system: HPLC (UV 254 nm) was coupled to GC using DB-17Ms capillary column (60 m × 0.25 mm i.d. × 0.15 μ), ion sources, quadrupole, 300°C, 200°C)	The compositional profile of PAHs across the olive oil samples showed a high abundance of PAHs of lower molecular weights and a large contribution of alkylated PAHs regardless of olive oil type	LOD and LOQ were reported, no validation data were reported; SIM reported, but selectivity was missing	[60]

Oleic acids (standard, crude, and pharmaceutical grades)	Identification and direct determination of fatty acid profile in oleic acid using HPLC-CAD and Ms-IT-TOF	Standard and samples were dissolved in ACN	HPLC-CAD coupled to Ms-IT-TOF; Dionex Acclaim 120 C_{18} column (4.6 × 250 mm, 5 μm), 35°C, gradient elution 0.5% glacial acetic acid and ACN; detailed CD and MS see original publication	27 fatty acids can be identified based on the exact mass by HR MS; The mean recovery values of all target analytes ranged from 96.5%–103.6%; RSD of repeatability and intermediate precision <5%, for components with concentrations > 0.05%	Linearity, LOD, LOQ, recovery, repeatability, and intermediate precision were reported. Peak identification was performed by HR-MS data	[61]
Edible vegetable oils	Rapid method for analysis of quantitative fatty acid profiles using UPLC-ESI-MS/MS	Oils in toluene (+ antioxidant butylated hydroxytoluene) derivatized using 2-dimethylami no ethanol	UPLC-ESI-MS/MS: Acquity UPLC BEH phenyl column (2.1 mm × 100 mm, 1.7 μm), 50°C, (A) 95% 10 mM NH_4Ac containing 5% ACN, B: ACN, Isocratic 90% B (2 min); MRM	By performing 1.5 min separation using the proposed method, accuracy: 93%–108% and precisions: 0.3%–2.0%., LOQ	Accuracy and precision were reported. Selectivity was not reported (confirmation of the peak identity using MRM)	[62]

(Continued)

Table 5.4 (Continued)

Samples	Issues	Sample preparation	LC conditions	Results	Validation	Ref.
Vegetables oils	Quantitative analysis of different lipid classes, lipid species, and regioisomers within the class	Oils dissolved in cyclohexane	HPLC-CAD; column: two Nucleodur C18 ISIS (250 × 2. 1 mm,1,8 μm, connected in series with a Security Guard ULTRA C18 (2.1 mm); column temperature programming and gradient elution	The proposed method can be applied to analyze complex lipid samples containing free fatty acids, fatty acid esters, mono acyl glycerides, TAG	Linearity, repeatability, and accuracy (standard addition) were reported; selectivity was not reported.	[63]
Oils extracted from sea buckthorn, (*Hippophaë rhamnoides* L. ssp. *mongolica*) grown in Finland	Stereospecific characterization of TAG using multidimen-sional-LC-MS	TAG fractions of the pulp oil samples were trans-esterified into fatty fatty acid methyl esters by a sodium methoxide	2 LC systems: HPLC-UV (205 nm) columns: achiral C18 for separation; LC-API-MS, using 2 CHIRALCEL OD-RH	The proposed method can be applied for revelation of stereospecific structural information of natural TAGs −impossible to obtain by other existed methods	No validation data were reported, including confirmation of the target peaks	[64]

Vegetables oils extracted from seed using Sep-Pak Cartridges Vac 35 cc	Separation of TAG containing allenic and acetylenic fatty acids by enantiomeric LC-MS	Oils were dissolved in an acetonitrile, propan-2-ol, hexane mixture (33:33:33% v/v/v).	LC-ESI-MS: LC column: 2 Astec Cyclobond I 2000 DMP (3,5-dimethyl-phenyl-carbamate modified β-cyclodextrin) chiral LC columns (5 μm, 25 cm × 4.6 mm) connected in series, details can be referred to in original publication	A total of six and three enantiomers of TAGs containing crepenynic and xi-menynic acids, respectively, were identified by chiral column analysis	Completed identification of the separated compounds were performed by comparing to standards (isolated or prepared)	[65]

2D-LC-APCI–MS, two-dimensional-liquid chromatography-atmospheric pressure chemical ionization; *HPLC-DAD*, high pressure liquid chromatography- diode array detector; *SPE*, solid phase extraction; *UPLC-ESI-MS/MS*, ultra-performance liquid chromatography-electrospray ionization-tandem mass spectrometry-mass spectrometry.

USP44-NF39 <852>; methods for qualification of the AAS (installation qualification (IQ), operational qualification (OQ), performance qualification (PQ)), procedure for preparation of standards/samples and validation/verifications are well described [66].

The essential requirements of any methods used at QC laboratory is cheap and fast, but it should be accurate and precise. New methods for quality assessment of fats and oils are constantly published in journals, and some of them have been discussed in previous sections. Therefore researchers at R&D laboratory need to develop more cheap, fast methods but yield similar to results of the existed validated methods. For this purpose, the researchers need to validate the proposed methods according to general chapter of USP-NF, namely, <1225> [24], <1210> [26], and <1010> [27] prior for routine applications.

It is well known that chemical profiling or chromatographic fingerprinting can be applied as a quality assessment tool for herbal drugs if the authentic botanical reference standards or standardized extracts or herbal preparations are available. Identical chromatographic fingerprints mean that the chemical compositions of sample and standard are similar (qualitatively and quantitatively) [52]. With the same concept, the chromatographic fingerprinting can be applied as a quality assessment tool for any edible fats and oils. The obtainability of an authentic fats or oils reference standard that meet all physical and chemical characterizations is described in each of their monograph pharmacopoeias are very crucial. The more sophisticated the chromatography instrument used, the more accurate the results, in this case the application of LC-HR-MS/MS is the best choice, but unfortunately this instrument maybe is too expensive. Further studies need to be performed to investigate whether the single analysis using chromatographic fingerprinting can replace all nonspecific and specific tests that are described in the monograph. Due to incapability of LC-HR-MS/MS methods for simultaneous analyzing organic and inorganic compounds, analysis samples using AAS still needs to be performed. The application of ion chromatography methods could be considered as the alternative method for analyzing the metals in fats and oils.

Acknowledgement

The authors wish to acknowledge Library of the University, Surabaya, Indonesia for awarding access to of the USP-NF online to GI.

References

[1] The United States Patent and Trademark Office (USPTO), CPC definition - subclass A23D. https://www.uspto.gov/web/patents/classification/cpc/html/defA23D.html, 2022 (accessed 20.03.22).

[2] S.P. Apte, Fixed-oil excipient monographs: development of USP fixed-oil reference standards, Pharmaceutical Technology. 37. https://www.pharmtech.com/journals/pharmaceutical-technology/pharmaceutical-technology-04-02-2013, 2013 (accessed 23.03.22).

[3] USP-NF, Hydrogenated vegetable oils. https://online.uspnf.com/uspnf/document/1_GUID-9385D882-A6E1-4D64-8DBE-FB959DF7DBEA_6_en-US, 2022 (accessed 23.03.22).

[4] A. Dieffenbacher, W.D. Pocklington, Standard Methods for the Analysis of Oils, Fats and Derivatives, 1St Supplement to the 7th Revised and Enlarged Edition, International Union of Pure and Applied Chemistry, Blackwell Scientific Publication, Oxford, London, Edinburg, Boston, 1992.

[5] USP-NF, USP45-NF40 <401> Fats and Fixed oils. https://online.uspnf.com/uspnf/document/1_GUID-DA3A8434-91C3-4E62-9AF4-33ED2BEE8369_4_en-US, 2022 (accessed 20.03.22).

[6] World Health Organization, Global Protocols for Measuring Fatty Acid Profile of Foods, with Emphasis on Monitoring Trans-fatty Acids Originating from Partially Hydrogenated Oils, Department of Nutrition and Food Safety, World Health Organization, Geneva, 2020.

[7] Ministry of Health and Family Welfare, Food Safety and Standards Authority of India, Manual of Methods of Analysis of Food, Oils and Fats (Revised), Ministry of Health and Welfare, Government of India, New Delhi, 2021.

[8] Y. Endo, Analytical methods to evaluate the quality of edible fats and oils: the JOCS standard methods for analysis of fats, oils and related materials (2013) and advanced methods, J. Oleo Sci. 67 (2018) 1–10. Available from: https://doi.org/10.5650/jos.ess17130.

[9] Metrohm USA Inc, Seven important parameters for analysis of edible oils and fats. https://www.news-medical.net/whitepaper/20190821/Seven-Important-Parameters-for-Analysis-of-Edible-Oils-and-Fats.aspx, 2019 (accessed 22.03.22).

[10] R.A. Moreau, Selected topics in the analysis of lipids. https://lipidlibrary.aocs.org/lipid-analysis/selected-topics-in-the-analysis-of-lipids, 2021 (accessed 22.03.22).

[11] International Olive Council (IOC), IOC standards, methods and guides. https://www.internationaloliveoil.org/what-we-do/chemistry-standardisation-unit/standards-and-methods/, 2022 (accessed 31.03.22).

[12] ISO, Standards by ISO/TC 34/SC 11. Animal and vegetable fats and oils. https://www.iso.org/committee/47936/x/catalogue/, 2022 (accessed 01.04.22).

[13] USP-NF, USP44-NF39 <202> Identification of fixed oils by thin-layer chromatography. https://online.uspnf.com/uspnf/document/1_GUID-17A1BCE5-269D-4CEC-8384-E4C81CD7AFC1_2_en-US, 2022 (accessed 01.03.22).

[14] H.E. Tahir, M. Arslan, G. Komla Mahunu, A. Adam Mariod, S.B.H. Hashim, Z. Xiaobo, et al., The use of analytical techniques coupled with chemometrics for tracing the geographical origin of oils: a systematic review (2013–2020, Food Chem. 366 (2022). Available from: https://doi.org/10.1016/j.foodchem.2021.130633.

[15] Council of Europe, European Pharmacopoeia Commission, European Directorate for the Quality of Medicines & Healthcare, European Pharmacopoeia, Tenth edition, 2019.

[16] L.C. Klein-Junior, M.R. de Souza, J. Viaene, T.M.B. Bresolin, A.L. de Gasper, A.T. Henriques, et al., Quality control of herbal medicines: from traditional techniques to state-of-the-art approaches, Planta Medica 87 (2021) 964–988. Available from: https://doi.org/10.1055/a-1529-8339.

[17] E. Reich, A. Schibli, Validation of high-performance thin-layer chromatographic methods for the identification of botanicals in a cGMP environment, n.d. https://academic.oup.com/jaoac/article/91/1/13/5656220.
[18] T.K.T. Do, I. Trettin, R. De Vaumas, S. Cañigueral, C. Valder, E. Reich, Proposal for a standardized method for the identification of essential oils by HPTLC, Pharmeuropa Bio & Scientific Notes, European Directorate for the Quality of Medicines & HealthCare (EDQM), Strasbourg, 2021.
[19] H. Ofori, D. Hettiarachchi, T. Sostaric, F. Busetti, M.C. Boyce, High-performance thin-layer chromatographic fingerprinting of sandalwood essential oils, J. Planar Chromatogr. Mod. TLC 32 (2019) 205–210. Available from: https://doi.org/10.1556/1006.2019.32.3.5.
[20] M. Srivastava, P. Maurya, S. Mishra, N. Kumar, K. Shanker, Chemotaxonomic differentiation of Clerodendrum species based on high-performance thin-layer chromatographic fingerprinting of key secondary metabolites and chemometric data analysis, J. Planar Chromatogr. Mod. TLC 32 (2019) 211–222. Available from: https://doi.org/10.1556/1006.2019.32.3.6.
[21] G. Alaerts, J. van Erps, S. Pieters, M. Dumarey, A.M. van Nederkassel, M. Goodarzi, et al., Similarity analyses of chromatographic fingerprints as tools for identification and quality control of green tea, J. Chromatogr. B: Anal. Technol. Biomed. Life Sci. 910 (2012) 61–70. Available from: https://doi.org/10.1016/j.jchromb.2012.04.031.
[22] M.R. Shen, Y. He, S.M. Shi, Development of chromatographic technologies for the quality control of Traditional Chinese Medicine in the Chinese Pharmacopoeia, J. Pharm. Anal. 11 (2021) 155–162. Available from: https://doi.org/10.1016/j.jpha.2020.11.008.
[23] R.S. Ibrahim, H.H. Zaatout, Unsupervised pattern recognition chemometrics for distinguishing different Egyptian Olive varieties using a new integrated densitometric reversed-phase high-performance thin-layer chromatography-image analysis technique, J. Planar Chromatogr. Mod. TLC 32 (2019) 453–460. Available from: https://doi.org/10.1556/1006.2019.32.6.2.
[24] USP-NF, USP44-NF39 <1225> Validation of compendial procedures. https://online.uspnf.com/uspnf/document/1_GUID-E2C6F9E8-EA71-4B72-A7BA-76ABD5E72964_4_en-US, 2022 (accessed 26.03.22).
[25] USP-NF, USP44-NF39 <1226> Verification of compendial procedures. https://online.uspnf.com/uspnf/document/1_GUID-18A6E56B-8EA7-4B37-AB7D-82352B73A309_3_en-US, 2022 (accessed 20.04.22).
[26] USP-NF, USP44-NF39 <1210> Statistical tools for procedure validation. https://online.uspnf.com/uspnf/document/1_GUID-13ED4BEB-4086-43B5-A7D7-994A02AF25C8_6_en-US, 2022 (accessed 23.01.22).
[27] USP-NF, USP44-NF39 <1010> Analytical data-interpretation and treatment. https://online.uspnf.com/uspnf/document/1_GUID-5C0818CD-E76F-44B8-B504-C202CA762F2A_5_en-US, 2022 (accessed 22.01.22).
[28] K. Ferenczi-Fodor, B. Renger, Z. Végh, The frustrated reviewer - recurrent failures in manuscripts describing validation of quantitative TLC/HPTLC procedures for analysis of pharmaceuticals, J. Planar Chromatogr. Mod. TLC (2010) 173–179. Available from: https://doi.org/10.1556/JPC.23.2010.3.1.
[29] G. Indrayanto, Validation of chromatographic methods of analysis: application for drugs that derived from herbs, Profiles of Drug Substances, Excipients and Related Methodology, Academic Press Inc, 2018, pp. 359–392. Available from: https://doi.org/10.1016/bs.podrm.2018.01.003.
[30] T. Hodisan, D. Casoni, M.S. Beldean-Galea, C. Cimpoiu, Identification and quantification of tocopherols in vegetable oils by thin-layer chromatography, J. Planar Chromatogr. Mod. TLC. 21 (2008) 213–215. Available from: https://doi.org/10.1556/JPC.21.2008.3.13.

[31] D. Demchenko, O.N. Pozharitskaya, A.N. Shikov, V.G. Makarov, Validated HPTLC method for quantification of vitamin D3 in fish oil, J. Planar Chromatogr. Mod. TLC 24 (2011) 487–490. Available from: https://doi.org/10.1556/JPC.24.2011.6.6.
[32] A. Zeb, M. Murkovic, High-performance thin-layer chromatographic method for monitoring the thermal degradation of β-carotene in sunflower oil, J. Planar Chromatogr. Mod. TLC 23 (2010) 35–39. Available from: https://doi.org/10.1556/JPC.23.2010.1.6.
[33] A. Lehri, J. Barthwal, A. Niranjan, D.V. Amla, Development and validation of hptlc densitometric method for identification and quantification of geraniol in palmarosa oil, J. Planar Chromatogr. Mod. TLC 24 (2011) 316–319. Available from: https://doi.org/10.1556/JPC.24.2011.4.8.
[34] M. Dabrowska, K. Sokalska, P. Gumulka, Z. Binert-Kusztal, M. Starek, Quantification of omega-3 fatty acids in dietary supplements and cooking products available on the polish market by thin-layer chromatography–densitometry, J. Planar Chromatogr. Mod. TLC 32 (2019) 13–24. Available from: https://doi.org/10.1556/1006.2019.32.1.2.
[35] B. Magnusson, U. Örnemark, Eurachem Guide, The fitness for purpose of analytical methods. https://www.eurachem.org/index.php/publications/guides/mv, 2014 (accessed 30.03.22).
[36] FDA Office of Regulatory Affair, ORA Laboratory Manual Volume II, ORA-LAB.5.4.5. https://www.fda.gov/media/73920/download, 2020 (accessed 21.10.21).
[37] Eur-Lex, Commission Implementing Regulation (EU) 2021/808, Official Journal of the European Union L180/84. https://eur-lex.europa.eu/legal-content/EN/TXT/?uri = CELEX%3A32021R0808, 2021 (accessed 31.03.22).
[38] USP-NF, USP44-NF39, Anise Oil. https://online.uspnf.com/uspnf/document/1_GUID-CABAB300-D3F0-4453-A34C-B728D6EB1B06_5_en-US, 2022 (accessed 30.03.22).
[39] H.D. Waktola, A.X. Zeng, S.T. Chin, P.J. Marriott, Advanced gas chromatography and mass spectrometry technologies for fatty acids and triacylglycerols analysis, TrAC. Trends Anal. Chem. 129 (2020). Available from: https://doi.org/10.1016/j.trac.2020.115957.
[40] M.F.S. Mota, H.D. Waktola, Y. Nolvachai, P.J. Marriott, Gas chromatography-mass spectrometry for characterisation, assessment of quality and authentication of seed and vegetable oils, TrAC. Trends Anal. Chem. 138 (2021). Available from: https://doi.org/10.1016/j.trac.2021.116238.
[41] Phenomenex, Analyzing Fats and Oils by GC. https://phenomenex.blob.core.windows.net/documents/b545a226-e776-4bab-8ec3-4ba45b926aaa.pdf, 2018 (accessed 05.04.22).
[42] Agilent CrossLab, Comprehensive Analysis of FAMEs, Fatty Acids, and Triglycerides, (n.d.). https://www.google.com/url?sa = t&rct = j&q = &esrc = s&source = web&cd = &ved = 2ahUKEwiR-abL4Pv2AhUuzTgGHbI5BXcQFnoECAMQAQ&url = http://www.agilent.com%2Fcs%2Flibrary%2Fbrochures%2F5991-8763EN_gc_fame_brochure.pdf&usg = AOvVaw3G3wlITf13SzxQ2DjqJiXG (accessed 05.04.22).
[43] J. Song, J. Park, J. Jung, C. Lee, S.Y. Gim, H.J. Ka, et al., Analysis of trans fat in edible oils with cooking process, Toxicol. Res. 31 (2015) 307–312. Available from: https://doi.org/10.5487/TR.2015.31.3.307.
[44] K. Pastor, V. Vujasinović, A.M. Jeromela, D. Vujić, D. Jovanović, M. Aćanski, Gas chromatography–mass spectrometry system applied to determine botanical origin of various types of edible vegetable oils, J. Serbian Chem. Soc. 84 (2019) 1017–1025. Available from: https://doi.org/10.2298/JSC180719109P.

[45] K. Yoshinaga, J. Obi, T. Nagai, H. Iioka, A. Yoshida, F. Beppu, et al., Quantification of triacylglycerol molecular species in edible fats and oils by gas chromatography-flame ionization detector using correction factors, J. Oleo Sci. 66 (2017) 259–268. Available from: https://doi.org/10.5650/jos.ess16180.
[46] A.L. Mihai, M. Negoi□ă, N. Belc, Evaluation of fatty acid profile of oils/fats by GC-MS through two quantification approaches, Rom. Biotechnol. Lett. 24 (2019) 973–985. Available from: https://doi.org/10.25083/rbl/24.6/973.985.
[47] T. Shi, G. Wu, Q. Jin, X. Wang, Detection of camellia oil adulteration using chemometrics based on fatty acids GC fingerprints and phytosterols GC–MS fingerprints, Food Chem. 352 (2021). Available from: https://doi.org/10.1016/j.foodchem.2021.129422.
[48] X. Wang, Y. Han, Y. Li, S. Wang, J. Wang, Detection of Qinghai-Tibet Plateau flaxseed oil adulteration based on fatty acid profiles and chemometrics, Food Control. 130 (2021). Available from: https://doi.org/10.1016/j.foodcont.2021.108332.
[49] P. Ioime, E. Piva, M. Pozzebon, J.P. Pascali, Automated sample preparation and analysis by gas chromatography tandem mass spectrometry (GC–MS/MS) for the determination of 3- and 2-monochloropropanediol (MCPD) esters and glycidol esters in edible oils, J. Chromatogr. A (2021)(1650). Available from: https://doi.org/10.1016/j.chroma.2021.462253.
[50] L. Zhao, T. Szakas, M. Churley, D. Lucas, Multi-class multi-residue analysis of pesticides in edible oils by gas chromatography-tandem mass spectrometry using liquid-liquid extraction and enhanced matrix removal lipid cartridge cleanup, J. Chromatogr. A 1584 (2019) 1–12. Available from: https://doi.org/10.1016/j.chroma.2018.11.022.
[51] E.P. de, P. Azevedo, E.M. dos Santos Alves, J.R.B. de Souza, K.S. de Araújo, S. de Santana Khan, et al., Fatty acid in raw and heated coconut oil in eleven coconut oil food preparations analysed by gas chromatography, Int. J. Gastronomy Food Sci. 24 (2021). Available from: https://doi.org/10.1016/j.ijgfs.2021.100329.
[52] G. Indrayanto, The importance of method validation in herbal drug research, J. Pharm. Biomed. Anal. 214 (2022) 114735. Available from: https://doi.org/10.1016/j.jpba.2022.114735.
[53] Gloria Márquez-Ruiz, Analysis of used frying oils and fats by high-performance size-exclusion chromatography. https://lipidlibrary.aocs.org/chemistry/physics/frying-oils/analysis-of-used-frying-oils-and-fats-by-high-performance-size-exclusion-chromatography, 2021 (accessed 15.04.22).
[54] Jean Louis Sébédio, William W. Christie, Analysis of trans polyunsaturated fatty acid. https://lipidlibrary.aocs.org/chemistry/physics/frying-oils/analysis-of-trans-polyunsaturated-fatty-acids, 2021 (accessed 15.04.22).
[55] G. Márquez-Ruiz, Determination of oxidized monomeric, dimeric and oligomeric triacylglycerols; diacylglycerols and free fatty acids. https://lipidlibrary.aocs.org/chemistry/physics/frying-oils/determination-of-oxidized-monomeric-dimeric-and-oligomeric-triacyl glycerols-diacylglycerols-and-free-fatty-acids, 2021 (accessed 15.04.22).
[56] F. Wei, N. Hu, X. Lv, X.Y. Dong, H. Chen, Quantitation of triacylglycerols in edible oils by off-line comprehensive two-dimensional liquid chromatography-atmospheric pressure chemical ionization mass spectrometry using a single column, J. Chromatogr. A 1404 (2015) 60–71. Available from: https://doi.org/10.1016/j.chroma.2015.05.058.
[57] A. Morales, S. Marmesat, M.V. Ruiz-Méndez, G. Márquez-Ruiz, J. Velasco, Formation of oxidation products in edible vegetable oils analyzed as FAME derivatives by HPLC-UV-ELSD, Food Res. Int. 62 (2014) 1080–1086. Available from: https://doi.org/10.1016/j.foodres.2014.05.063.

[58] J. Velasco, A. Morales-Barroso, M.V. Ruiz-Méndez, G. Márquez-Ruiz, Quantitative determination of major oxidation products in edible oils by direct NP-HPLC-DAD analysis, J. Chromatogr. A 1547 (2018) 62–70. Available from: https://doi.org/10.1016/j.chroma.2018.03.014.
[59] L. Wang, J. Wang, J. Xu, S. Liu, S. Huang, S. Han, et al., Highly sensitive qualitative and quantitative detection of saturated fatty aldehydes in edible vegetable oils using a "turn-on" fluorescent probe by high performance liquid chromatography, J. Chromatogr. A 1621 (2020). Available from: https://doi.org/10.1016/j.chroma.2020.461063.
[60] H. Ekner, K. Dreij, I. Sadiktsis, Determination of polycyclic aromatic hydrocarbons in commercial olive oils by HPLC/GC/MS—occurrence, composition and sources, Food Control. 132 (2022). Available from: https://doi.org/10.1016/j.foodcont.2021.108528.
[61] X. Zhao, Y. He, J. Chen, J. Zhang, L. Chen, B. Wang, et al., Identification and direct determination of fatty acids profile in oleic acid by HPLC-CAD and MS-IT-TOF, J. Pharm. Biomed. Anal. 204 (2021). Available from: https://doi.org/10.1016/j.jpba.2021.114238.
[62] S.K. Nagumalli, C.C. Jacob, G. Gamboa da Costa, A rapid and highly sensitive UPLC-ESI-MS/MS method for the analysis of the fatty acid profile of edible vegetable oils, J. Chromatogr. B: Anal. Technol. Biomed. Life Sci. 1161 (2020). Available from: https://doi.org/10.1016/j.jchromb.2020.122415.
[63] A. Causevic, K. Olofsson, P. Adlercreutz, C. Grey, Non-aqueous reversed phase liquid chromatography with charged aerosol detection for quantitative lipid analysis with improved accuracy, J. Chromatogr. A 1652 (2021). Available from: https://doi.org/10.1016/j.chroma.2021.462374.
[64] M. Kalpio, K.M. Linderborg, M. Fabritius, H. Kallio, B. Yang, Strategy for stereospecific characterization of natural triacylglycerols using multidimensional chromatography and mass spectrometry, J. Chromatogr. A 1641 (2021). Available from: https://doi.org/10.1016/j.chroma.2021.461992.
[65] A. Palyzová, T. Řezanka, Separation of triacylglycerols containing allenic and acetylenic fatty acids by enantiomeric liquid chromatography-mass spectrometry, J. Chromatogr. A 1623 (2020). Available from: https://doi.org/10.1016/j.chroma.2020.461161.
[66] USP-NF, USP44-NF39 <852> Atomic Absorption Spectroscopy. https://online.uspnf.com/uspnf/document/1_GUID-7A2010E3-BE15-4F5F-9D2B-FA3C47F69220_2_en-US, 2021 (accessed 15.11.21).

CHAPTER SIX

Gas chromatography and multivariate analysis for wheat flours

Prinya Wongsa[1] and Nithiya Rattanapanone[2]
[1]Food Science and Technology Program, School of Agro-Industry, Mae Fah Luang University, Chiang Rai, Thailand
[2]Department of Food Science and Technology, Faculty of Agro-Industry, Chiang Mai University, Chiang Mai, Thailand

6.1 Introduction

Wheat (*Triticum* spp.) is an important cereal grain providing macromolecules and energy for human nutrition and is used as a staple food and animal feed. They are cultivated in tropical and subtropical areas, requiring fertile soil and a temperate climate. In 2010, the world production of wheat was 640.1 million tonnes grown in 215.6 million hectares, while the global production in 2020 was 760.1 million tonnes planted in 219.0 million hectares [1]. Major wheat growing countries include China, India, Russia, United States, France, Australia, Canada, Pakistan, Ukraine, and Germany.

The genus *Triticum* of the family Gramineae (grass family) consists of many species of wheat including einkorn (*Triticum monococcum*), emmer (*Triticum dicoccum*), spelt (*Triticum spelta*), common or club wheat (*Triticum aestivum*), and durum wheat (*Triticum durum*). Some ancient varieties of wheat including einkorn, emmer, and spelt are still being cultivated for special purposes, while common wheat is the most important and widely cultivated of all wheat species [2]. Modern wheat varieties can be classified according to seed time (spring/winter), hardness (soft/hard), and color (white/red) [3]. According to wheat hardness, there are three major categories of wheats including hard, soft, and durum wheat varieties due to a different in their protein contents. The protein contains ranged from 10%–14% and 8%–11% for hard and soft wheat, respectively [4,5]. Protein content is one of the most important quality factors in wheat and varies widely depending on the cultivar, agronomic, and climatic conditions.

Food Quality Analysis.
DOI: https://doi.org/10.1016/B978-0-323-95988-9.00008-4

Flours milled from soft wheat kernels are whiter in color and finer to the touch than hard wheat flours. Therefore, hard wheat flours are considered strong flours, and soft wheat flours form weak gluten and are sometimes called weak flours

The classification based on color refers to the color of the aleurone or outer layer of the wheat kernel. In general, there are six categories of wheat, namely, hard red winter, hard red spring, soft red winter, durum, soft white, and hard white wheat [3].

Wheat flour is widely used for human consumption. A total of 55% of processed wheat flour is estimated to be used in the baking and confectionery industry, 17% is used for domestic consumption, 15% for dough, 11% for cookies, and 2% for the production of drugs, glue, and animal feeding [6]. In addition, common wheat flour is used in making wheat-based foods, such as breads, doughnuts and cakes [4], while durum wheat is used in most dried pasta and couscous. Asian foods including white salted and yellow alkaline noodles, instant noodles, and steamed bread and dumplings also require wheat of different quality [7].

6.2 Wheat grain compositions

Grain of common wheat contains 2%–3% DM germ, 13%–17% dried matter (DM) bran, and 80%–85% endosperm [8]. The chemical compositions of wheat grain consist of starch (60%–68%), protein (7%–18%), moisture (8%–18%), lipids (1.5%–2%), cellulose (2%–2.5%), and ash (1.5%–2%) [9]. In addition, grain of common wheat acts as a source dietary fiber, vitamin E phenolic compounds, carotenoids, tocopherols, alkylresorcinols, γ-oryzanols, dietary fibers, and β-glucans [10]. Ferulic acid was the major phenolic acid found in wheat flour, followed by syringic and *p*-hydroxybenzoic acids found in wheat flour [11]. Black wheat variety had the highest total phenolic content (659.8 μg gallic acid equivalents/g) and total flavonoid content (319.3 μg rutin equivalents/g), whereas light purple wheat had the lowest total flavonoid content (236.2 μg rutin equivalents/g). In addition, the highest phenolic acids were found in flours of winter wheat (1171 μg/g) with average levels of 658 μg/g total phenolics across all of the wheat genotypes [12]. Whole wheat flour and partially debranned grain flour had significantly higher total phenolic contents, total flavonoid contents, and antioxidant activity than refined flour.

Potential health benefits of whole grains wheat are attributed to bioactive metabolites including phenolic acids, flavonoids, and phytosterols. Flavonoids possess anti-inflammatory, antioxidant, antiallergic, antithrombotic, antiviral, and anticarcinogenic activities [13]. Regular daily intake of whole grain products is associated with reduced risk of several diseases [14]. However, the relationship between the Western diet based on wheat-based products and lifestyle and health outcomes, and the increasing prevalence of obesity, type 2 diabetes, and allergy and food intolerances have been observed [2]. Furthermore, specific proteins are responsible for triggering hypersensitivities such as wheat allergy, celiac disease (CD) and nonceliac gluten sensitivity (NCGS) [15].

6.3 Wheat flour

The AACC International has defined "whole wheat flour" as the product obtained by grainding from wheat kernels (other than durum). Therefore, it consists of bran, germ, and endosperm components [16]. In addition, wheat flour is the product prepared from grain of common wheat by grinding or milling processes in which the bran and germ are partly removed and the remainder is comminuted to a suitable degree of fineness [17].

The two predominant techniques for grinding whole grain flours are stone and roller mills [18]. White flour is derived from the starchy endosperm storage tissue of the grain and mainly comprises starch (75%–85%), water (14%), protein (10%–12%), and lipids (2.0%–2.5%) [19,20].

Besides starch, protein is the major constituent of wheat flour. Gluten is a storage protein found in cereal grains including barley, rye, wheat, and oats. It is an insoluble protein mainly composed of glutenins and gliadins [21]. Gluten provides the viscoelastic properties of dough that characterizes texture of breads and cakes. Flour from hard varieties derived from common wheat contains high gluten content and is preferred in bakery products. The hardest-kernelled wheat is durum macaroni wheat; it is essential for manufacturing pasta products. Gluten was detected by using different types of ELISA test kits at 24.0–40.2 g/kg in bread, 6.5–72.6 g/kg in noodles, and 23.0–86.9 g/kg in different powder food samples including corn starch, green bean powder, potato starch, rice starch [22]. The difference in milling caused by variation in plate, hammer, stone, roller mills, etc., affected protein and lipid composition of whole wheat flour protein and lipid composition of strong and weak wheat flour. Loss of total amino acids was observed in all-milled flour. Unsaturated fatty acid content including linolenic acid was lower in stone-milled flour (1.3%), followed by plate mill (2.2%), hammer mill (2.8%), and roller flour mill (3.8%) [23].

6.4 The standard for wheat flour

Quality characteristics of wheat are determined by different physiochemical and rheological analysis by using different methods recommended by AACC [24]. In addition, the CODEX ALIMENTARIUS has set up the international standard for wheat flour CXS 152−1985 [17] and the European Commission (EC) has issued the maximum contamination levels (MCLs) for a range of mycotoxins (aflatoxins, ochratoxin A, patulin, deoxynivalenol, and zearalenone) for various food products including wheat [25]. The MCLs set by EC for common commercial mycotoxins including Deoxynivalenol (DON), Zearalenone (ZEA), and Ochratoxin A (OTA) in cereals are 750 μg/kg, 75 μg/kg, and 3 μg/kg, respectively.

6.5 Quality assessment of wheat and wheat-based products

In order to assure a quality and safety of wheat and wheat-based products, conventional and nondestructive applications for monitoring and detection quality of products have been implemented.

In addition, the wheat and wheat-based industries apply analytical practices in order to monitor and control quality of their products. The conventional methods include starch gelatinization, hydration, dough resistance, dough strength particle charge detection, GlutoPeak, and solvent retention [26].

Nondestructive applications include visible and near-infrared spectroscopy, a rapid, safe, and precise method used to monitor and quantify protein, gluten, moisture content, and starch in some wheat varieties treated by different nitrogen fertilization rates [27,28]. In addition, noninvasive techniques such as Fourier transform infrared (FTIR) spectroscopy,

Raman spectroscopy, and multivariate analysis techniques, for example, principal component analysis (PCA) and/or partial least square discrimination analysis (PLS-DA) can help discriminate and classify the substitution and adulteration of wheat flour with cheaper cereals including barley, rye, and spelt [29]. PCA loading plots revealed that the discrimination was based on an assessment of protein signals and changes in starch, protein, and arabinoxylan signals. The application of FITR spectroscopy coupled with multivariate analysis has been used for identifying wheat varieties. Using FTIR spectrum, the intensity of absorbance of moisture, protein, fat, ash, carbohydrates, and hardness of grain were determined [30]. The discrimination of the spectra was primarily based on starch, protein, and arabinoxylan signals. In addition, PCA and PLS analysis showed a clear differentiation of the species with accuracies greater than 98% [31].

6.6 Application of gas chromatography coupled with mass spectroscopy

Gas chromatography (GC) is a type of chromatographic technique, which, according to the International Union of Pure and Applied Chemistry (IUPAC) recommendation, is defined as a separation technique in which the mobile phase is a gas [32].

GC is always carried out in a separated column. It is a separation and detection method for sample mixtures whose components can be volatilized without thermal decomposition. This technique is used to separate mixtures of gaseous chemical compounds based on differences in the compounds' relative affinities for a solid (gas—solid chromatography) or liquid (gas—liquid chromatography) stationary phase held within a column [33].

GC technique is used in the laboratories of the chemical, petrochemical, and pharmaceutical industries, research institutes, as well as in the clinical, environmental, and food and beverage analyses. Recent developments in GC have resulted in the introduction of better and selective fused silica capillary columns and methods for sample preparation. Moreover, newer separation and detection solutions, such as fast GC, multidimensional separation GC techniques (GC × GC), and hyphenation of GC and GC × GC with mass spectrometry (MS), with triple quadrupole MS and with time-of-flight MS (TOF-MS), have been developed and become industrial routine.

In addition, multidimensional gas chromatography (MDGC) consists of more than one column with different selectivity. The connection of the automated sample preparation techniques with MDGC and detector results in quantitative and qualitative analysis of a wide variety of sample matrices for analytes at parts per billion (ppb) concentrations.

Hyphenated gas chromatography referred to the coupling of the high-performance separation technique of gas chromatography in order to obtain information-rich and sophisticated GC detectors, which can be operated as a stand-alone instrument for chemical analysis and enhanced automated online sample preparation systems. The current hyphenated GC techniques include GC–MS, GC-FTIR, and GC nuclear magnetic resonance (GC-NMR) for detection of molecular analytes as well as Gas chromatography - Atomic Absorption Spectroscopy (GC-AAS) and Gas chromatography-Atomic Emission Spectroscopy (GC-AES) coupling for elemental analysis [34]. In addition, hyphenated gas chromatography involves coupling of the GC to automated sample preparation techniques including solid-phase microextraction (SPME), large-volume injection (LVI), purge and trap (PT), and headspace (HS).

GC–MS instrument is composed of at least the following two major devices including a gas chromatograph and a mass spectrometer. Chemical compounds' mixtures are injected and separated into individual components in a column in the GC. Consequently, the individual compound is introduced and converted into ions, identified, and/or quantified at a molecular level in the mass spectrometer. At the same time, highly specific nature of a mass spectrum makes the mass spectrometer a very specific GC instruments [35].

Owing to its high spread capacity and robustness, GC–MS is a commonly employed technique, typically implemented in food quality control, quality assurance, and metabolomics study. It is used for the qualitative and quantitative analysis for food compositions, flavors and aroma compositions, food additives, food adulterants, and contaminants such as pesticides and toxin [36].

In addition, GC–MS-based metabolomics is used in (1) studying metabolites in plants and animal tissues, which can provide metabolite profile; (2) metabolite fingerprinting, which that separates or verifies food and can be very useful to obtain new insights into human, plant, and microbial biochemistry; (3) drug and biomarker discovery; (4) nutrition research; and (5) food control [37].

6.6.1 Gas chromatography coupled with mass spectroscopy analytical procedures

Prior to GC–MS analysis, the analyzed compounds can be classified in two groups. The first group consists of nonvolatile compounds including disaccharides, polyphenols, and lipophilic compounds. These compounds require specific analytical treatment, including derivatization for their analysis by GC. The second group comprises volatile and semivolatile compounds. These compounds do not require any derivatization.

The analysis of volatile organic compounds (VOCs) is one of the most accurate and efficient techniques. The vaporized analytes are carried through by the inert heated mobile phase or carrier gas such as helium. The separation of vaporized mixtures occurs in the capillary column.

6.6.1.1 Extraction techniques

Sample preparation is the basic and most crucial step for the success of any analytical method. Sample pretreatment techniques include solid–liquid extraction (SLE), liquid–liquid extraction (LLE), and solid-phase extraction, while analytical techniques of volatile compounds can be carried out using headspace (HS) methods including dynamic headspace (DHS), static headspace (SHS), and HS–SPME.

Conventional solvent extraction including SLE and LLE of samples is carried out by using organic solvents such as MeOH: H_2O and ethanol are still used for sample preparation and extraction of polar compounds, bioactive compounds or polyphenols including alkaloids, cardiac glycosides, flavonoids, phenols, phlobatannin, reducing sugars, saponins, steroids, tannins, terpenoids, volatile oils, carbohydrates, and protein/amino acids in plants [38].

HS method is defined as the vapor phase formed above solid or liquid when it is heated within a sealed vial, establishing an equilibrium between the molecules that have escaped to the gas phase and the solid or liquid phase (matrix sample) [39]. In DHS sampling, the volatile fraction is recovered from the gaseous flow stream stripped through (purge-and-trap approach) or over (dynamic approach) the matrix onto a suitable trapping system (e.g., cold trap) or medium (a sorbent, an adsorbent, or a specific reagent or solvent for a specific class or classes of compounds). In addition, in SHS sampling, the liquid or solid sample sealed in the HS vial is equilibrated at a given temperature for a suitable time; at equilibrium, an aliquot of the resulting vapor phase is transferred to the GC system for analysis.

In addition, SPME is a new sample preparation technique that uses a fused-silica fiber coated on the outside with an appropriate stationary phase, an (ad)sorbent layer. Analyte in the sample is directly extracted to the fiber coating [40]. Commercial coatings for SPME including dimethylpolysiloxane, polyacrylate, Carboxen, carbowax, and divinylbenzene (DVB) in different combinations are available in the market. The fused silica fiber can be inserted into the gaseous or liquid sample to carry out analysis of the HS or by direct immersion (DI), respectively. After exposure for a certain period of time of the fiber in the sample until the equilibrium is reached, the fiber is retracted, and the SPME needle is desorbed in the hot inlet of the GC to carry out sample analysis.

6.6.1.2 Derivatization

Derivatization prior to GC-MS is an essential preparatory step to change the analyte properties including reduction in polarity and increase in volatility, and thermal stability of metabolites [41–43].

In GC–MS, derivatization reaction includes alkylation (e.g., methylation), formation of aryl derivatives, silylation (e.g., formation of trimethylsilyl derivatives), acylation (e.g., reactions with acyl chlorides or with chloroformates), and several other types of derivatizations [41]. Alkylation involves the replacement of the hydrogen of the polar groups in the analytes, for example, –OH, –SH, –NH–, –COOH, –CONH–, with alkyl groups to yield more volatile ethers, thioethers, N-alkyl amines, esters, and N-alkyl amides, respectively. The principal alkylation reagents include diazomethane, tetraalkylammonium (TAA) salts, alcohols (acid as catalyst), and alkyl halides. Among these, TAA salts have acquired more popularity due to their high reaction rate, high derivatization efficiency, and operation convenience [44]. In silylation reaction, trimethylsilyl (TMS), the most applicable trialkylsilyl derivatization reagent, reacts with a wide range of oxyanions to form thermally stable derivatives. Silyl derivatives are probably the most widely used derivatization reagents employed in GC [44]. In addition, acylation is used to prepare acylated derivatives for NH–, –OH, and –SH groups using carboxylic acid, acid anhydride, acyl halide, and activated acyl amide as derivatization reagents [45]. Acylation with acid anhydride requires the use of anhydrous conditions to avoid hydrolysis of the reagent.

6.6.1.3 Chromatographic techniques

In GC–MS, the driving force for the separation is the distinguishable interactions of analytes with the stationary phase and the mobile phase.

Analytical conditions including the column's dimensions (length, diameter, film thickness), type of carrier gas, column temperature (gradient), as well as the properties of the stationary phase (e.g., alkylpolysiloxane) influence the efficiency and performance of GC and GC–MS. During elution, different analytes spend different time (retention time) in the GC column due to their different adsorption rates on the stationary phase or different partition between the mobile phase (carrier gas) and the stationary phase (of a capillary column in gas–liquid chromatography). Consequently, the separated analyte flow further into the MS through an interface. This is followed by ionization, mass analysis, and detection of mass-to-charge ratios of ions generated from each analyte by the mass spectrometer. The combination of GC and MS provides a much accurate chemical identification than either technique used separately [34]. In addition, metabolites are identified using GC–MS by comparing with databases such as Wiley and NIST 14 library of volatile compounds.

6.6.1.4 GC–MS data processing and statistical analysis

Generally, GC–MS and GC–MS-based metabolomics approaches generate large multivariate data sets, which are common in the food research area and require sophisticated analytical tools to analyze [46,47]. In addition, a high-throughput data processing workflow includes feature detection and alignment, data reduction, and spectral-matching-based annotation [48]. Typically, univariate and multivariate statistics are applied in the analyses of data analysis, depending on the type of experiments performed. The univariate analysis including *t*-test and one-way analysis of variance provides a preliminary overview of the data's characteristic potential for discrimination. In food sciences, multivariate data analysis (MVDA) is generally used to deal with the authenticity, classification, discrimination, fraud and origin of foods.

MVDA concerns two learning methods, namely, unsupervised and supervised data analysis [47–49]. Unsupervised approaches attempt to divide the data set into groups without any predefined categorization of the samples where patterns or trends among samples are defined during the analysis, without a priori knowledge of the patterns or groups. PCA and hierarchical cluster analysis (HCA) are the two most commonly used unsupervised methods. PCA is used to determine the differences or similarities between the samples observed. However, supervised methods are based on a priori assignment of objects or samples into class memberships for the creation of a respective mathematical model (e.g., training set).

Afterward, unknown objects (e.g., test set or validation) could be predicted based on the models generated. Discriminant analysis including Partial least square discrimination analysis (PLS-DA), and Orthogonal projections to latent structures discrimination analysis (OPLS-DA) is a supervised method used for discrimination of samples or variables and describes the classification information in one component.

In addition, the development, growth, and incorporation of food systems in the global economy relies on better and improved methods for the analysis of foods. The application of different tools or methodologies allowed for quality control processes, regulatory enforcement activities, and problem-solving tasks that are based on the application of modern statistics concepts, experimental design, and chemometrics, where they have become an integral part of the analytical process and analysis of foods [50,51]. By definition, "chemometrics" is the chemical discipline that uses mathematical, statistical, and other methods employing formal logic to design or select optima and use measurement procedure and experiment to provide maximum relevant chemical information by analyzing chemical data [52]. Therefore, complementary disciplines and tools such as statistics, experimental design, and chemometrics have become essential in modern sciences and are an integral component in quality analysis of food products.

6.7 Application of gas chromatography coupled with mass spectroscopy and multivariate analysis in quality analysis of wheat flour and wheat-based products

GC–MS and GC–MS-based metabolomics combined with multivariate analysis or chemometrics have recently been applied in the evaluation of the natural variance apparent in chemical and metabolite compositions.

6.7.1 Gas chromatography coupled with mass spectroscopy in analysis of wheat components/chemical composition

Comparison types of flour including wheat, spelt, and pseudocereals (amaranth and buckwheat) with respect to the content of carbohydrates was carried out by using GC–MS chromatography and chemometric tools. Cereal flour was defatted with hexane. Carbohydrates were derivatized by using TMSI (trimethylsilylimidazole) to obtain trimethylsilyl ethers. Sugar components including pentoses, hexoses, and disaccharides were identified using 73 and 217 Da mass and the library search. The cluster analysis showed that buckwheat, wheat, spelt, and amaranth are three separate branches with four groups. PCA indicated that spelt and amaranth are indistinguishable, while wheat and buckwheat were well separated and grouped [53].

6.7.2 Gas chromatography coupled with mass spectroscopy analysis of volatile organic compounds in wheat flour and wheat-based products

VOCs have a great influence on aroma attribute and consumer acceptability of food products. In addition, VOC analysis is a useful tool in classification and authentication processes. In a study, 72 compounds in whole meal of 81-different wheat varieties and landraces were extracted by dynamic HS extraction and analyzed using GC–MS. Multivariate analysis of the data showed a large diversity in volatile profiles between samples. Principal components obtained from PLS-DA on the volatile profile data showed a differentiation between wheat-growing regions. In addition, dissimilarity of landraces and modern wheat varieties was observed on their volatile profiles. Landraces had higher levels of esters, alcohols, and some furans, while modern varieties contained higher levels of terpenes, pyrazines, and straight-chain aldehydes [54].

Wheat was classified according to its origin by analysis of their VOCs. Six wheat cultivars harvested in different areas was extracted using SPME and analyzed based on GC–MS. The GC–MS analysis identified 158 VOCs. PCA and PLS of VOCs showed the discrimination of wheat samples based on their origin (species and area of cultivation) [55].

In addition, Riccardo De Flaviis et al. analyzed the VOC profile of common and durum wheat kernels grown in different fields sited at different altitudes over two years and identified 149 compounds using GC–MS. PCA suggested that environmental conditions were more important than species in the determination of the VOC's variance of wheat.

Wheat varieties cultivated in different sites were characterized by distinctive VOC profiles, and many compounds including odor-active compounds were used to classify wheat based on its origin [56].

The cultivars of durum wheat were distinguished on its volatile fraction by using the extraction of HS–SPME and the analytical method of GC–MS. Eleven different chemical classes including alcohols and aldehydes, acids, alkanes, aromatic, and heterocyclic hydrocarbons were observed. PCA showed that cultivars were well separated. Anco Marzio was characterized by nonanal, 2-nonenal, butanol, and acetophenone, while Sculptur was characterized by dodecane, 2-heptanone, 6-methyl-2-heptanone, 2-undecanone, tridecane, and 2-propanol [57].

The VOCs or bread in flour-based fermentation produced by yeast strains was studied by using GC–MS and chemometric tools. PLS analysis indicated that the VOC including 3-methyl-1-butanol, 2-phenylethyl alcohol, nonanal, and benzaldehyde were closely related with the whole wheat flour, while 2-methyl-1-propyl acetate, and 2-methyl-1-propanol were observed to be correlated with the fermentation temperature. PCA showed that fermentation temperature was related to the accumulation of benzaldehyde and nonanal. Extending the fermentation time increased alcohol and ester accumulation. Therefore, bread-related volatiles produce was related to yeast strains and fermentation conditions of wheat flour [58].

Heat treatment has been applied to tailoring the functional properties of flour. Heat treatment conducted at 140°C–160°C for 15–60 min can also improve binding and thickening properties of various cereal flours, which provides the potential to replace chemically cross-linked starches. The application of heat-treated flour in foods helps in the elimination of microorganisms contained in raw flour and improvement of functional properties of flour. However, heat treatment influences volatile compounds and modifies sensory characteristics of flour. Volatile fingerprints obtained from GC–MS showed that the untreated waxy wheat flour contained higher levels of odor-active compounds than normal wheat flour including aldehydes, alcohols, furans, and ketones. Low-heat temperature (100°C–110°C) treatments eliminated cereal odor (aldehyde), while heat treatments at 120°C and higher temperatures increased the content of pyrazines, furans, and sulfur-containing compounds, which gave a roasty aroma to the flours [59].

6.8 Gas chromatography coupled with mass spectroscopy-based metabolomics in wheat study

Metabolomics science involves studying for a global understanding of biological systems. Metabolomics approaches including GC–MS, liquid chromatography mass spectrometry (LC–MS), capillary electrophoresis mass spectrometry (CE–MS), and Fourier transform infrared spectrometry

(FTIR) approaches have been applied and provide the potential in advancement of health, environmental, and food science research [46,60,61]. GC–MS-based metabolomics approaches provide wide coverage of compound classes including organic and amino acids, sugars, sugar alcohols, phosphorylated intermediates, and lipophilic compounds [46].

Untargeted GC–MS based metabolomic analysis was performed to study the response to high-nitrogen fertilizer during wheat grain development. The application of high-nitrogen fertilizer resulted in a significant increase in wheat biomass, grain number, and yield, and improved flour quality in terms of protein and gluten content, dough rheological properties, and starch and bread-making quality. Metabolite profiling obtained from six wheat grain development identified 74 metabolites, including amino acids, carbohydrates, organic acids, and lipids/alcohols. These frist metabolites are primarily involved in carbon and nitrogen metabolisms. Moreover, two principal components (PC1 and PC2) reported the main variances caused by nitrogen-fertilizer treatment. The high-nitrogen treatment mediated a significant accumulation of metabolites involved in the TCA cycle, starch, and protiens [62].

Genotype, environment, and genotype-by-environment interactions influence the metabolite profile of durum wheat grain. In a study, four durum wheat cultivars were grown under conventional and organic farming systems over three consecutive years. GC–MS platform identified a large group of metabolites, including amino acids, sugars, sugar alcohols, and organic acids, together with other metabolites such as phytosterols, tocopherols, and fatty acids. The PCA score plots show that the higher and lower contents of each metabolite of durum wheat samples were positively and negatively correlated with PC1. PC1 discriminated durum wheat samples that came from growing seasons, and PC2 allowed very clear differentiation of the agronomic system Moreover, statistical analysis of the data showed a small impact of genotype and large effects of both year and genotype-by-environment interaction on the metabolite composition and quality of the wheat grain [63].

Identification of biomarkers enables to distinguish organic and conventional wheat flour. Metabolites were extracted using methanol and analyzed by GC–MS. There were 48 metabolites, and 245 nonidentified metabolites were detected. PCA showed a sample clustering according to farming systems and significant differences in peak areas between the farming systems. Results obtained from all 11 cultivars indicated a greater influence of the cultivar than the farming system on metabolite concentrations. Based on individual cultivars, metabolite profiling showed promising results for the classification of organic and conventional wheat [64].

6.9 Gas chromatography coupled with mass spectroscopy wheat authentication

The authentication of food products is essential for food quality and safety. Authenticity assessments are important to ensure that the ingredients or contents of food products are legitimate and safe to consume. The authentication of food may affect many deceptive processes, such as the mislabeling of its origin, techniques of production, or forms of technical processing such as irradiation, freezing, and microwave heating. Nowadays, many efficient chemical analytical technologies and instruments including GC, LC, FTIR, NMR, and MS have been used to identify and detect emerging fraudulent trends in various food samples [65,66]. Vibrational spectroscopy analyses such as near infrared spectroscopy and FTIR spectroscopy in combination with multivariate data analysis methods, such as PCA and/or PLS-DA show potential in wheat authenticity to discriminate geographical origin, cultivar/classification and offer many advantages such as being user-friendly, cost-effective, time-saving, and environment-friendly [67].

An increase in demand of a staple food including wheat and wheat flour is observed and results in the substitution and adulteration of grains with cheaper cereals. Cereals, pseudocereals, flours, and bread, as mostly used bakery products in human nutrition, are usually differentiated according to varietal, botanical, or geographical origin by combining GC analysis with chemometric processing of the obtained data. The chemical compounds that have the role of discriminating factors usually involve small molecules, such as simple soluble sugars and free fatty acids. Analytical approaches based on the measurement of multiple markers and/or complex chemical or physical profiles/fingerprints supported by multivariate statistical analysis seem more promising in this respect [68].

GC methods are successfully applied in the authentication of flours of a wider spectra of plant species (cereals and some pseudocereals) used in bread-making.

In a study, GC–MS was used to perform a qualitative analysis of the liposoluble flour extract of different types of cereals (bread wheat and spelt) and pseudocereals (amaranth and buckwheat). Trimethylsulfonium hydroxide (TMSH) was used as a trans-esterification reagent. The liposoluble extract contained fatty acids, higher hydrocarbons, and phytosterols. Cluster analysis was applied to compare the liposoluble flour extract from different types of cereals and pseudocereals and enabled determination of flour origin [69].

In addition, Pastor et al. investigated the possibility of chemical differentiation between small grain flour including wheat, barley, oat, triticale, rye, and corn flour samples by using GC/MS and multivariate data analysis [70]. All cereal flour samples were defatted with hexane and extracted with ethanol. Extracted simple sugars (monosaccharides, disaccharides, trisaccharides, and sugar alcohols) were analyzed in the form of their corresponding trimethylsilyl oximes. With the application of principal coordinate analysis and HCA to obtain data, samples of corn flour were clearly distinguished from all samples of small grain flour.

6.10 Gas chromatography coupled with mass spectroscopy in wheat and wheat-based food spoilage and storage

Storage conditions of wheat also influence on the quality properties of wheat varieties. Temperature is one of the most important environmental factors for grain storage. The crude protein, hectoliter weight, thousand grain weights, Zeleny sedimentation, wet gluten, and dry gluten decreased at different rates according to changes in the grain moisture content [71] Moreover, pathogen's control on wheat and wheat flour is an important safety issue [72].

In addition, volatile compounds are used as an indicator of fungal activity at the early quality changes in cereal grains. The range of volatiles produced by spoilage fungi in vitro and on grain. The key volatile compounds indicated spoilage of grain during storage [73]. Moreover, lipids are a minor component in wheat flour, and their concentration and composition indicate the quality properties of wheat final products. Lipids are easily degraded during storage, which is the main cause of quality loss. The enzymatic degradation of lipids is carried out by the activation of endogenous and/or fungal enzymatic activities, which produce hydrolytic and oxidative rancidity. The volatile compounds produced by oxidative rancidity are the main indicators of deterioration [74]. Monitoring of lipid rancidity can be carried out by using GC−MS technique.

In a study, stored wheat grain was analyzed by using HS analysis combined with gas chromatography flame ionization detection and GC−MS for the production of VOCs by postharvest fungi by determining the production of VOCs. GC−MS identified three VOCs including cyclooctasiloxane, hexadecamethyl, produced by *Alternaria alternata*, and pentadecane produced by *A. infectora*. These compounds were observed at both the early and later stages of fungal growth. Therefore, fungal VOCs may be useful for early detection of postharvest fungi in grain, prior to the occurrence of visual symptoms [75].

Identification of the VOCs released by insects can be used to detect insects in stored grains. VOCs including methyl-1,4-benzoquinone; ethyl-1,4-benzoquinone; and 1-tridecene, released by *Tribolium castaneum* (red flour beetle) and *Cryptolestes ferrugineus* (rusty grain beetle), was detected by using headspace and GC–MS analysis [76].

6.11 Future gas chromatography coupled with mass spectroscopy application in wheat food safety

Food safety is a field of utmost importance in food science and technology. Awareness toward the microbial quality of wheat has been raised due to the food-borne illness and outbreaks associated with contaminated wheat flour [72].

There has been an increase in application of GC–MS and/or GC–MS-based metabolomics approaches to detect of totally or partially forbidden compounds sought, determine potentially dangerous compounds (e.g., pollutants and toxins) or organisms that could be present in food and might pose a risk for consumers' health [77]. Pesticides have played a very important role in the development of the agriculture. Chemical hazards of pesticides have led to the attention of food safety and human health. A multiresidue method for the determination of 24 pesticides in wheat, white flour, and bran using GC–MS with negative chemical ionization and selected ion monitoring was developed and validated. The QuEChERS, which stands for quick, easy, and cheap method was used for the extraction of different pesticides [78]. The QuEChERS multiresidue procedure omits or replaces many complicated analytical steps commonly employed in traditional methods by easier ones. However, the application of multivariate analysis on GC–MS chromatographic data is still limited.

6.12 Conclusions

Gas chromatograph coupled with multivariate analysis, an instrument and statistical technique used in most analytical laboratories and research institutes worldwide, can be successfully applied in compound analysis, authentication, and fraud detection procedures of various food and beverage products, such as wheat and wheat-based products. It can be concluded that application of GC and GC–MS with multivariate analysis in further development of metabolomics approaches for authentication and safety could provide us with meaningful results, thus representing a significant contribution to this emerging field in the future.

References

[1] FAOSTAT. *FAO statistics* 2020, Available from <https://www.fao.org/faostat/en/2022> (accessed 01.12.21).

[2] P.R. Shewry, Do ancient types of wheat have health benefits compared with modern bread wheat? J. Cereal Sci. 79 (2018) 469–476.

[3] P. Rosenfelder, M. Eklund, R. Mosenthin, Nutritive value of wheat and wheat by-products in pig nutrition: a review, Anim. Feed. Sci. Technol. 185 (s3–4) (2013) 107–125.

[4] N. Caporaso, M.B. Whitworth, I.D. Fisk, Protein content prediction in single wheat kernels using hyperspectral imaging, Food Chem. 240 (2018) 32–42.

[5] J.A. Delcour, I.J. Joye, B. Pareyt, E. Wilderjans, K. Brijs, B. Lagrain, Wheat gluten functionality as a quality determinant in cereal-based food products, Annu. Rev. Food Sci. Technol. 3 (2012) 469–492.

[6] M.C. Ferrari, M.T.P.S. Clerici, Y.K. Chang, A comparative study among methods used for wheat flour analysis and for measurements of gluten properties using the wheat gluten quality analyser (WGQA), Food Sci. Technol. Camp. 34 (2) (2014) 235–242.

[7] G.B. Crosbie, S. Huang, I.R. Barclay, Wheat quality requirements of Asian foods, Euphytica 100 (1998) 155–156.

[8] Z. Šramková, E. Gregová, E. Šturdík, Chemical composition and nutritional quality of wheat grain, Acta Chim. Slov. 2 (1) (2009) 115–138.

[9] Matz S.A. 1991. The Chemistry and Technology of Cereals as Food and Feed, (2nd ed.). Springer, New York, USA.

[10] D.L. Luthria, Y. Lu, K.M.M. John, Bioactive phytochemicals in wheat: extraction, analysis, processing, and functional properties, J. Func. Food 18 (2015) 910–925.

[11] L. Hernández, D. Afonso, E.M. Rodríguez, C. Díaz, Phenolic compounds in wheat grain cultivars, Plant Foods Hum. Nutr. 66 (2011) 408–415.

[12] L. Li, P.R. Shewry, J.L. Ward, Phenolic acids in wheat varieties in the HEALTHGRAIN diversity screen, J. Agric. Food Chem. 56 (21) (2008) 9732–9739.

[13] P.R. Shewry, S.J. Hey, The contribution of wheat to human diet and health, Food Energy Secur. 4 (3) (2015) 178–202.

[14] P.K. Chachaiya, G. Mehta, Evaluation of secondary metabolites in wheat grain (Triticum Sp.) grown in humid south eastern plain zone of Rajasthan (India), Int. J. Agric. Environ. Biotechnol. 12 (3) (2019) 249–260.

[15] K. Schalk, B. Lexhaller, P. Koehler, K.A. Scherf, Isolation and characterization of gluten protein types from wheat, rye, barley and oats for use as reference materials, PLoS One 12 (2) (2017) e0172819. Available from: https://doi.org/10.1371/journal.pone.0172819.

[16] AACC International, 1999. AACC International defines whole grain. Available from: <http://aaccnet.org/definitions/wholegrain.asp> (accessed 01.12.21).

[17] FAO and WHO. The CODEX ALIMENTARIUS international food standard. Standard for wheat flour CXS 152–1985. 2019. Rome Italy.
[18] A.F. Doblado-Maldonado, O.A. Pike, J.C. Sweley, D.J. Rose, Key issues and challenges in whole wheat flour milling and storage, J. Cereal Sci. 56 (2012) 119–126.
[19] B. Min, I. González-Thuillier, S.J. Powers, P. Wilde, P.R. Shewry, R.P. Haslam, Effects of cultivar and nitrogen nutrition on the lipid composition of wheat flour, J. Agric. Food Chem. 65 (2017) 5427–5434.
[20] H. Goesaert, K. Brijs, W.S. Veraverbeke, C.M. Courtin, K. Gebruers, J.A. Delcour, Wheat flour constituents: how they impact bread quality, and how to impact their functionality, Trends Food Sci. Technol. 16 (2005) 12–30.
[21] J.R. Biesiekierski, What is gluten? J. Gastroenterol. Hepatol. 32 (Suppl. 1) (2017) 78–81.
[22] J.M. Yu, J.H. Lee, J.-D. Park, Y.-S. Choi, J.-M. Sung, H.W. Jang, Analyzing gluten content in various food products using different types of ELISA test kits, Foods 10 (2021) 108. Available from: https://doi.org/10.3390/foods10010108.
[23] P. Prabhasankar, P.H. Rao, Effect of different milling methods on chemical composition of whole wheat flour, Eur. Food Res. Technol. 213 (2001) 465–469.
[24] AACC. 2000. Approved methods of the AACC. The American Association of Cereal Chemists, St. Paul.MN.US.
[25] European Commission 2006. COMMISSION REGULATION (EC) No 1881/2006 of 19 December 2006 setting maximum levels for certain contaminants in foodstuffs. Official Journal of the European Union.
[26] R.M. Amir, F.M. Anjum, M.I. Khan, M.R. Khan, I. Pasha, M. Nadeem, Wheat four quality evaluation from the baker's perspective: comparative assessment of 18 analytical methods, Eur. Food Res. Technol. 244 (2018) 535–545.
[27] A. Ibrahim, A. Csúr-Varga, M. Jolánkai, H. Mansour, A. Hamed, Monitoring some quality attributes of different wheat varieties by infrared technology, Agric. Eng. Int. 20 (1) (2018) 201–210.
[28] V. Cortés, J. Blasco, N. Aleixos, S. Cubero, P. Talens, Monitoring strategies for quality control of agricultural products using visible and near-infrared spectroscopy: a review, Trends Food Sci. Technol. 85 (2019) 138–148.
[29] J. Kniese, A.M. Race, H. Schmidt, Classification of cereal flour species using Raman spectroscopy in combination with spectra quality control and multivariate statistical analysis, J. Cereal Sci. 101 (2021) 103299.
[30] R.M. Amir, F.M. Anjum, M.I. Khan, M.R. Khan, I. Pasha, M. Nadeem, Application of Fourier transform infrared (FTIR) spectroscopy for the identification of wheat varieties, J. Food Sci. Technol. 50 (5) (2013) 1018–1023.
[31] K. Sujka, P. Koczon', A.C. Nska, M. Reder, Ciemniewska-gytkiewicz H. The application of FT-IR spectroscopy for quality control of flours obtained from Polish producers, J. Anal. Methods Chem. 2017 (2017) 4315678. Available from: https://doi.org/10.1155/2017/4315678.
[32] Todd J.F.J. Recommendations for nomenclature and symbolism for mass spectroscopy (including an appendix of terms used in vacuum technology) (IUPAC recommendations 1991). Pure Appl. Chem., 1991 63(10), 1541-1566, <https://www.degruyter.com/database/IUPAC/entry/iupac.63.0090/html> (Accessed on 14 January 2022).
[33] Kusch P. Introductory chapter: gas chromatography – the most versatile analytical technique, in: Gas Chromatography – Derivatization, Sample Preparation, Application. IntechOpen. 2019; Available from: https://doi.org/10.5772/intechopen.73339.
[34] Guo X., Lankmayr E. Hyphenated techniques in gas chromatography. In Advanced Gas Chromatography – Progress in Agricultural, Biomedical and Industrial Applications. Mustafa Ali M.(Ed.). IntechOpen 2012; Available from: https://doi.org/10.5772/2518.

[35] K. Chaturvedi, R.K. Nanda, Hyphenated gas chromatography, Int. J. Pharm. Sci. Rev. Res. 5 (3) (2010) 18–27.
[36] A. Chauhan, M.K. Goyal, P. Chauhan, GC-MS technique and its analytical applications in science and technology, J. Anal. Bioanal. Tech. 5 (2014) 222. Available from: https://doi.org/10.4172/2155-9872.1000222.
[37] M. Vinaixa, E.L. Schymanski, S. Neumann, M. Navar, R.M. Salek, O. Yanes, Mass spectral databases for LC/MS- and GC/MS-based metabolomics: state of the field and future prospects, TrAC. Trends Anal. Chem. 78 (2016) 23–35.
[38] L.K. Kanthal, A. Dey, K. Satyavathi, P. Bhojaraju, GC-MS analysis of bio-active compounds in methanolic extract of Lactuca runcinata DC, Pharmacogn. Res. 6 (1) (2014) 58–61.
[39] J. Pico, M. Gómez, J. Bernal, J.L. Bernal, Analytical methods for volatile compounds in wheat bread, J. Chromatogr. A 1428 (2016) 55–71. Available from: https://doi.org/10.1016/j.chroma.2015.09.045.
[40] H. Kataoka, H.L. Lord, J. Pawliszyn, Applications of solid-phase microextraction in food analysis, J. Chromatogr. A 880 (1–2) (2000) 35–62.
[41] Moldoveanu S.C., David V. Derivatization methods in GC and GC/MS. In Gas Chromatography – Derivatization, Sample Preparation, Application. Kusch P.(Ed.). IntechOpen 2019; Available from: https://doi.org/10.5772/intechopen.73339.
[42] J. Rohloff, Analysis of phenolic and cyclic compounds in plants using derivatization techniques in combination with GC-MS-based metabolite profiling, Molecules 20 (2015) 3431–3462. Available from: https://doi.org/10.3390/molecules20023431.
[43] Qiu Y., Reed D. Gas chromatography in metabolomics study. Advances in Gas Chromatography. Xinghua G. (Ed.). IntechOpen. 2014; Available from: https://doi.org/10.5772/57397.
[44] S.G. Villas-Bôas, K.F. Smart, S. Sivakumaran, G.A. Lane, Alkylation or Silylation for analysis of amino and non-amino organic acids by GC-MS? Metabolites 1 (2011) 3–20. Available from: https://doi.org/10.3390/metabo1010003.
[45] A.I. Ruiz-Matute, O. Hernández-Hernández, S. Rodríguez-Sánchez, M.L. Sanz, I. Martínez-Castro, Derivatization of carbohydrates for GC and GC–MS analyses, J. Chromatogr. B 879 (2011) 1226–1240.
[46] J. Lisec, N. Schauer, J. Kopka, L. Willmitzer, A.R. Fernie, Gas chromatography mass spectrometry–based metabolite profiling in plants, Nat. Protoc. 1 (1) (2006) 387–396.
[47] C. Buve', W. Saeys, M.A. Rasmussen, B. Neckebroeck, M. Hendrickx, T. Grauwet, et al., Application of multivariate data analysis for food quality investigations: an example-based review, Food Res. Int. 151 (2022) 110878.
[48] L. Yao, A.M. Sheflin, C.D. Broeckling, J.E. Prenni, Data processing for GC-MS- and LC-MS-based untargeted metabolomics, Methods Mol. Biol. c1978 (2019) 287–299. Available from: https://doi.org/10.1007/978-1-4939-9236-2_18.
[49] N. Doyle, D. Swain, J.J. Roberts, D. Cozzolino, The use of qualitative analysis in food research and technology: considerations and reflections from an applied point of view, Food Anal. Methods 10 (2017) 964–969.
[50] J.J. Roberts, D. Cozzolino, An overview on the application of chemometrics in food science and technology—an approach to quantitative data analysis, Food Anal. Methods 9 (2016) 3258–3267.
[51] N. Feizi, F.S. Hashemi-Nasab, F. Golpelichi, N. Saburouh, H. Parastar, Recent trends in application of chemometric methods for GC-MS and GC × GC-MS-based metabolomic studies, Trends Anal. Chem. 138 (2021) 116239.
[52] K. He'berger, Chemoinformatics- multivariate mathematical-statistical methods for data evaluation, in: T. Ka'roly Ve'key Andea's, V. Akos (Eds.), Medical Application of Mass Spectrometry, Elservier B.V, 2008.

[53] M.A. Ačanski, D.N. Vujic, Comparing sugar components of cereal and pseudocereal flour by GC−MS analysis, Food Chem. 145 (2014) 743−748.

[54] G. Starr, M.A. Petersen, B.M. Jespersen, S. Hansen, Variation of volatile compounds among wheat varieties and landraces, Food Chem. 174 (2015) 527−537.

[55] R. De Flaviis, G. Sacchetti, D. Mastrocola, Wheat classification according to its origin by an implemented volatile organic compounds analysis, Food Chem. 341 (2021) 128217.

[56] R. De Flaviis, D. Mutarutwa, G. Sacchetti, D. Mastrocola, Could environmental effect overcome genetic? A chemometric study on wheat volatiles fingerprint, Food Chem. 372 (2022) 131236. 2022.

[57] E. Mattiolo, F. Licciardello, G.M. Lombardo, G. Muratore, U. Anastasi, Volatile profiling of durum wheat kernels by HS−SPME/GC−MS, Eur. Food Res. Technol. 243 (2017) 147−155.

[58] R. Niçin, N. Özdemir, Ö. Şimşek, A. HilmiÇon, Production of volatiles relation to bread aroma in flour-based fermentation with yeast, Food Chem. 378 (2022) 132125.

[59] J. Xu, W. Zhang, K. Adhikari, Y.-C. Shi, Determination of volatile compounds in heat-treated straight-grade flours from normal and waxy wheats, J. Cereal Sci. 75 (2017) 77−83.

[60] A.-H.M. Emwas, N. Al-Rifai, K. Szczepski, S. Alsuhaymi, S. Rayyan, H. Almahasheer, et al., You are what you eat: application of metabolomics approaches to advance nutrition research, Foods 10 (2021) 1249. Available from: https://doi.org/10.3390/foods10061249.

[61] M. Fraga-Corral, M. Carpena, M.A. Garcia-Oliveira, J. Simal-Gandara, Analytical metabolomics and applications in health, environmental and food science, Crit. Rev. Anal. Chem. 52 (4) (2022) 712−734. Available from: https://doi.org/10.1080/10408347.2020.1823811.

[62] S. Zhen, J. Zhou, X. Deng, G. Zhu, H. Cao, Z. Wang, et al., Metabolite profiling of the response to high-nitrogen fertilizer during grain development of bread wheat (Triticum aestivum L.), J. Cereal Sci. 69 (2016) 85−94.

[63] B. Romina, P. Cristiano, N. Franca, V. Pasquale De, C. Luigi, P. Roberto, Effect of genotype, environment and genotype-by-environment interaction on metabolite profiling in durum wheat (Triticum durum Desf.) grain, J. Cereal Sci. 57 (2013) 183−192.

[64] A. Bonte, H. Neuweger, A. Goesmann, C. Thonar, P. Mader, G. Langenkämper, et al., Metabolite profiling on wheat grain to enable a distinction of samples from organic and conventional farming systems, J. Sci. Food Agric. 94 (2014) 2605−2612.

[65] J. Salamat, N.A.A. Rozani, S. Murugesu, Application of the metabolomics approach in food authentication, Molecules 26 (2021) 7565. Available from: https://doi.org/10.3390/molecules26247565.

[66] Pastor K., Ačanski M., Vujić D. Gas chromatography in food authentication. Gas Chromatography – Derivatization, Sample Preparation, Application. Kusch P.(Ed.). IntechOpen. 2019; Available from: https://doi.org/10.5772/interchopen.73339.

[67] Liu H.-Y., Wadood S.A., Xia Y., Liu Y., Guo H., Guo B.-L., et al. Wheat authentication: an overview on different techniques and chemometric methods. Crit. Rev. Food Sci. Nutr. 2021; July 1: 1−24. Available from: https://doi.org/10.1080/10408398.2021.1942783.

[68] E. E Capuano, R. Boerrigter-Eenling, G. van der Veer, S.M. Ruth, Analytical authentication of organic products: an overview of markers, J. Sci. Food Agric. 93 (2013) 12−28.

[69] M.A. Ačanski, D.N. Vujić, P.B. Psodorov, Practical method for the confirmation of authentic flours of different types of cereals and pseudocereals, Food Chem. 172 (2015) 314−317.

[70] K. Pastor, M. Ačanski, D. Vujić, G. Bekavac, S. Milovac, S. Kravić, Rapid method for small grain and corn flour authentication using GC/EI–MS and multivariate analysis, Food Anal. Methods 91 (2016) 443–450.
[71] H. Kibar, Influence of storage conditions on the quality properties of wheat Varieties, J. Stored Prod. Res. 62 (2015) 8–15.
[72] A.M.M. Lo'pez, S. Simsek, Pathogen's control on wheat and wheat flour: a review, Cereal Chem. 98 (1) (2020) 17–30.
[73] N. Magan, P. Evans, Volatiles as an indicator of fungal activity and differentiation between species, and the potential use of electronic nose technology for early detection of grain spoilage, J. Stored Prod. Res. 36 (4) (2000) 319–340.
[74] T.M. Alconad, M.C. Moure, Deterioration of lipids in stored wheat grains by environmental conditions and fungal infection – a review, J. Stored Prod. Res. 95 (2022) 101914.
[75] E.H. Barkat, B. Du, Y. Ren, G.E.St.J. Hardy, K.L. Bayliss, Volatile organic compounds associated with postharvest fungi detected in stored wheat grain, Australasian Plant Pathol. 46 (2017) 483–492.
[76] T. Senthilkumar, D.S. Jayas, N.D.G. White, M.S. Freund, C. Shafai, D.J. Thomson, Characterization of volatile organic compounds released by granivorous insects in stored wheat, J. Stored Prod. Res. 48 (2012) 91–96.
[77] M. Castro-Puyana, R. Pérez-Míguez, L. Montero, M. Herrero, Application of mass spectrometry-based metabolomics approaches for foodsafety, quality and traceability, Trends Anal. Chem. 93 (2017) 102–118. Available from: https://doi.org/10.1016/j.trac.2017.08.007.
[78] D.I. Kolberg, O.D. Prestes, M.B. Adaime, R. Zanella, Development of a fast multiresidue method for the determination of pesticides in dry samples (wheat grains, flour and bran) using QuEChERS based method and GC–MS, Food Chem. 125 (2011) 1436–1442.

CHAPTER SEVEN

Electrochemical sensors coupled with machine learning for food safety and quality inspection

Gabriella Magarelli[1,2], Alessandra Maia Freire[1,3] and Luciano Paulino Silva[1,3]

[1]Laboratory of Nanobiotechnology (LNANO), Embrapa Genetic Resources and Biotechnology, Brasilia, Distrito Federal, Brazil
[2]Laboratory of Food Safety (LSA), Embrapa Genetic Resources and Biotechnology, Brasilia, Distrito Federal, Brazil
[3]University of Brasilia (UnB), Brasilia, Distrito Federal, Brazil

7.1 Introduction

Food safety refers to all those hazards (e.g., chemical, biological, or physical), whether chronic or acute, that may make food potentially injurious to the health of consumers. Food production chains present multiple possibilities for food contamination to occur. Food production, processing, distribution, and transport, and preparation, with the added pressure of food globalization, all contribute to over 200 distinct known food-borne diseases and illnesses. The rigorous control concerning the quantities of chemical additives in food and beverages, the food-borne diseases caused by microorganisms, and the chemicals from polluted food or water have emerged as vital for food industries and for consumers. This increasing interest has promoted the urgency of improving and applying analytical food quality control systems along the whole food production chain, not only at the end of the process, searching for systems with more robust, faster, and reliable performances typically achieved by coupling information technology tools [1–3].

Rapid and accurate analysis of food is essential to screen for agents that may cause expressive health risks as pathogens, allergens, toxins, pesticides, chemical additives, antibiotic residues, and heavy metals. These biological and chemical contaminants can occur throughout each food production chain and can be associated with several key factors, including: environmental

Food Quality Analysis.
DOI: https://doi.org/10.1016/B978-0-323-95988-9.00001-1

issues, such as the presence of pollutants in the air, soil, and water; characteristics of the food raw materials, such as the natural presence of microorganisms or hazardous, noxious, and toxic substances in plants and animals; or technologies and inputs used in production, which can change substances present in foods into forms exhibiting hazardous potential or transfer compounds with such potential [4]. Most of the time, contamination can be avoided or reduced by adopting proper agricultural and production practices. In fact, the focus of good production practices is to minimize this risk. However, there are situations in which the complete elimination of the contaminant is impossible, unfeasible, or tiny amounts of these agents can be tolerated without causing considerable harm to health. In such cases, maximum acceptable limits are established, which usually vary by type of food and intake. Limits must be based on analytical principles and grounded in the protection of human health. Foods with contaminant levels higher than those recommended in the regulations cannot be sold. The World Health Organization (WHO) and the United Nations Food and Agriculture Organization (FAO), recognized worldwide by experts and foreign health authorities, have developed science-based risk assessments to define safe exposure levels to contaminants, which form the basis for the development of national and international food safety standards to protect the health of the consumers and ensure locally and globally accepted fair trade practices [4]. To this end, it is vital to adopt powerful analytical methods with high selectivity and sensitivity to detect food contaminants with the potential to reduce the adverse impacts that food contamination has on people. Conventional analytical methods based on techniques like gas chromatography (GC), high-performance liquid chromatography (HPLC), mass spectrometry (MS), enzyme-linked immunosorbent assay (ELISA), surface-enhanced Raman spectroscopy (SERS), ultraviolet–visible (UV–visible) spectroscopy, or fluorescence spectroscopy have been widely used for detecting food contaminants [5]. However, these methods overall share several limitations of being laborious, expensive, time-consuming, requiring large sample volumes, and involving highly trained personnel. The added cost makes these methods and instruments most suitable in academic and industrial settings rather than in-field measurements.

Chromatographic techniques can be used as powerful tools for quantitative analysis of organic food contaminants as pesticides, mycotoxins, or other small-molecule compounds that contaminate food sources, leaving out bacteria, proteins, and other larger food contaminants [5]. ELISA is considered the gold standard for the detection of small molecules, proteins, and bacterial food, but it cannot detect multiple contaminants at the same time. Furthermore, the development of a novel ELISA and other immunoassays can be expensive and take months due to the time needed for generating, synthesizing, and purifying the desired antigens and antibodies for specific sensing. Multiple food contaminants are frequently found on a single food source and further chemometric analysis or other data processing is often needed to distinguish between multiple signals on targets or differentiate the target from a matrix. In such respect, SERS is extremely useful for analyzing pathogens and toxins but often requires additional analysis, especially in complex food matrices, where the spectra may be very complicated, making it less desirable for real-world applications [5]. UV − visible spectroscopy is a useful and effective technique for food contaminant detection but may fail in terms of selectivity. In fact, the presence of a food matrix can mask the absorption peak due to other small molecules in solution that can absorb in the same UV or visible wavelength or larger matrix components that may nonspecifically scatter UV − visible light [5].

To overcome the disadvantages of traditional analytical techniques related to high cost, lack of portability, and offer real-time assessment throughout the food production chain, the adoption of sensors and biosensors are considered reliable strategies. These devices can rapidly measure the presence of toxic contaminants in food so that remediation actions can be taken [6]. Indeed, sensors offer a possible alternative by allowing screening of food samples for any potential contaminants before the production process is complete [7]. These systems can offer the possibility of rapid, on-site monitoring, and real-time information. In this chapter, electrochemical sensors and biosensors will be presented as possibilities to overcome the challenges of other analytical techniques mainly when integrated with information technology tools aiming to enhance the performance of the methods. Analytical methods using electrochemical sensors have achieved prominence in food safety analysis as an alternative to more traditional techniques like chromatography and MS. The most noteworthy advantages of electrochemical (bio)sensors are sensitivity, low limits of detection, large dynamic range, selectivity, linearity, fast response time, no/simplified sample preparation, and stability [2].

Otherwise, many authors consider electrochemical (bio)sensors not ideal for on-site food safety recognition if compared to optical sensors mainly because electrochemical strategies present higher complexity when requiring special tools to read the results. Despite this consideration, electrochemical (bio)sensors have shown a lower limit of detection (LoD) for detection of several food contaminants than optical sensors [8]. Currently, there is a possible direction for the integration of electrochemical strategies involving the use of bioreceptors, metal nanoparticles, carbon-based nanomaterials, and/or metal–organic frameworks (MOFs) with simpler sensing electrochemical devices as paper-based analytical devices [9]. At last, sustainable challenges must be addressed in the field of food safety analysis such as minimizing or eliminating sample preparation and obtaining high accuracy and reproducibility of the method in order to facilitate the transition of the developed (bio)sensors from the laboratory to their commercialization. Biosensors with antibodies or aptamers as bioreceptors restrict the biosensors to short shelf-life and poor stability. Seeking to overcome the limitations of the use of biosensors, researchers have been looking for innovative alternatives such as the use of machine learning (ML) to analyze and even predict sensing data [10]. Given the amount of large data required for ML applications, sensor analytical performance is of great importance, and their designs should consider measurements with repeatability and long lifetime, although this also depends on the target being analyzed and the functional material of the sensor system [11]. In (bio)sensors, the presence of interference affects the sensor's performance, and ML helps in removing signals obtained from the contaminants to obtain high sensitivity [12].

7.2 Electrochemical sensor types used in food science and technology

Chemical sensors consist of a transduction element covered with a chemical or biological recognition layer. This layer interacts with the target analyte, and the chemical changes resulting from this interaction are translated by the transduction element to electrical signals [9]. Electrochemical sensors represent an important subclass of chemical sensors in which an electrode is used as the transduction element [13]. The reactions under investigations typically generate a measurable current (amperometric sensor), a measurable potential (potentiometric sensor), a measurable conductivity (conductometric sensor), or a measurable impedance related to resistance and reactance (impedimetric sensor), as shown in Fig. 7.1. In the case of voltammetric sensors, analyte data can be obtained by varying the potential and subsequently measuring the resulting current

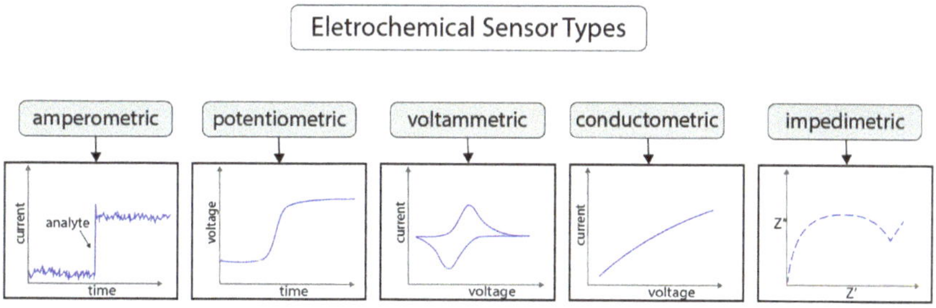

Figure 7.1 Electrochemical sensor types and their typical signals.

(Fig. 7.1). In a voltammogram, the intensity of a peak is directly proportional to the concentration of the analyte. The way the potential is applied defines the voltammetric technique, such as linear sweep (cyclic voltammetry) differential pulse voltammetry, and square wave voltammetry [14]. Electrochemical impedance spectroscopy (EIS) measures the effective resistance of an electrical circuit in response to the application of a sinusoidal alternating current (AC) potential with a small excitation amplitude. Amperometric detection is based on measuring the current generated by redox reactions involving the analyte at the electrode surface under a given potential. The linear relationship between the analyte concentration and the measured current can be established. Electrochemical techniques involve a reference, an auxiliary, and a working electrode. Reference electrodes often composed of silver−silver chloride (Ag−AgCl) provide a stable potential, independent of the sample composition, against which the potential of the working electrode is compared. An inert conducting material, such as platinum wire or graphite is typically used as the current-carrying in electrochemical cell. The working electrode, at which the reaction of interest occurs, acts as the transducer [12,15].

Some modern electrochemical (bio)sensors have been developed specifically for the detection of food contamination, including impedimetric aptasensors, square wave voltammetric electrodes, amperometric electrodes, and field-effect transistors. Electrochemical biosensors combine the analytical power of electroanalytical techniques with the specificity of a biologically sensitive recognition element such as antibodies, nucleic acids, enzymes, organelles, whole cells, and aptamers, which can be immobilized on an electrochemical transducer, and connected to a detector [16] (Fig. 7.2). Over the last 10 years, a considerable growth in the field of electrochemical biosensors for food safety analysis was observed, mainly due to the development of novel biorecognition molecules, such as

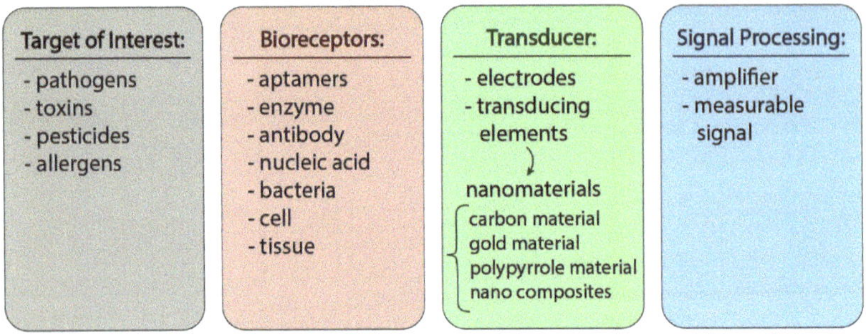

Figure 7.2 Scheme of principal components in food biosensors.

synthetic aptamers, DNA, cells, and bacteria and the recent developments of nanomaterial synthesis and nanotechnology field [7,12,14].

An interesting feature in electrochemical (bio)sensors for food safety analysis is the application of portable screen-printed electrodes (SPEs), which are electrochemical measurement devices manufactured by printing different types of ink (e.g., carbon, silver, gold, platinum) on paper, polymeric, or ceramic substrates. The composition of the different inks and the possibility of modifying inks by adding different enzymes, metallic nanoparticles, carbon nanotubes, polymers, or complexing agents determines its selectivity and sensitivity. These portable electrochemical sensors are good alternatives to facilitate the screening of potentially contaminated samples remotely at food production and handling areas where the resources are limited and specialized equipment are not available [6,17].

Nanoscale-developed food sensors are of recent interest as they improve electrochemical and electronic properties by increasing the surface area-to-volume ratio for sensitive reading out signals, increasing the electronic surface charge transfer, and adding catalytic properties. Several nanostructured materials, including conductive polymers (polypyrrole, chitosan, PEDOT), metal–metal oxide, carbon-based materials, quantum dots, and nanocomposite materials have been used to develop active platforms of nanosensor devices for food assessment [3,18,19]. Electrochemical detection systems based on SPEs have already been integrated with nanostructures in nanotechnology-based sensing approaches providing benefits as immobilization support for biomolecules, mediator to promote electron transfer reaction, and catalyst to amplify the electrochemical signal (Fig. 7.3). The introduction of nanostructured-materials for surface modification or as transducer elements has also improved analytical parameters such as sensitivity and LoD [9,20]. Currently, an increasing number of

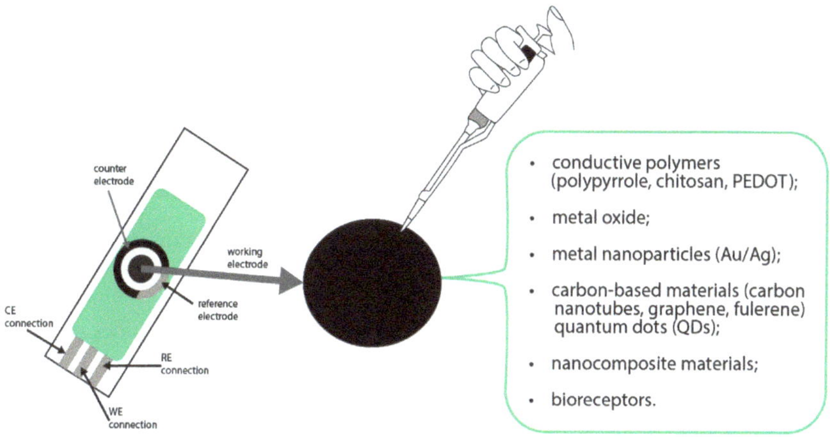

Figure 7.3 Portable electrochemical sensors and their nanostructured interface.

reports are being published on electrochemical (bio)sensors for the detection of food contaminants including pathogens, allergens, toxins, pesticides, chemical additives, antibiotic residues. and heavy metals [14,21].

Electrochemical immunosensors and electrochemical aptasensors are efficient platforms that have been extensively developed for the detection of food bacteria pathogens, (e.g., *Listeria monocytogenes*, *Escherichia coli* O157:H7, *Staphylococcus aureus*, and *Salmonella enterica*), mycotoxins (e.g., aflatoxin and ochratoxin A, zearalenone, fumonisin, and tricotecenos), and allergens (e.g., glycoproteins (antigens), cell-mediated (nonimmunoglobulin E [non-IgE]) or mixed IgE/cell-mediated) [21–23]. Electrochemical immunosensors and electrochemical aptasensors offer several advantages over the standard conventional methods such as ELISA, polymerase chain reaction (PCR), HPLC–MS, and surface plasmon resonance for detection of bacterial pathogens, mycotoxins, and allergens, which require considerable amounts of laboratory equipment, consumables, time, and trained personnel [7,23–25]. Some food contaminants are summarized in Table 7.1.

In electrochemical immunosensors, the bioreceptors are antibodies (Ab), also called immunoglobulins (Ig), which are large Y-shaped glycoproteins that can recognize an antigen (molecules capable of stimulating an immune response) typically with a high specificity [26]. In electrochemical aptasensors, the bioreceptors are aptamers, which are oligonucleotide chains (single-strain DNA or RNA), or peptides, which adopt a three-dimensional conformation in the space that has a very high affinity for a specific target molecule specifically bound to it [7,26]. These sensors

Table 7.1 Summary of food contaminants.

Foodborne pathogens	• Food-borne pathogens are the source of over 200 diseases leading annually to over 420,000 deaths worldwide • The most common symptom of food-borne illness is diarrhea, although severe symptoms may occur such as renal failure, liver failure, central nervous system disorders, reactive arthritis, cancer, and even death [24] • The most common food-borne diseases are those caused by *Listeria monocytogenes*, *Escherichia coli* O157:H7, *Staphylococcus aureus*, and *Salmonella enterica* • The complete list of pathogenic food bacteria includes many other pathogens [26]
Toxins	• Toxins in foods have become an important factor affecting food safety • The main sources of food-related toxins are those compounds existing in food itself and the toxins produced by some microorganisms in the process of food production and processing due to improper operation [27] • Some typical mycotoxins are mainly produced by *Aspergillus* (aflatoxin and ochratoxin A), *Penicillium* (ochratoxin A), or *Fusarium* (zearalenone, fumonisin, and tricotecenos toxins), which have severe toxic effects on humans, including hepatotoxicity, carcinogenicity, and nephrotoxicity • Mycotoxins can contaminate a range of foods, like milk, coffee, grains, beer, and grape juice. There are several other toxins in foods already mentioned in other publications [28]
Allergens	• Food allergies are mainly related to allergen-specific IgE-mediated immune hypersensitivity, usually for some food proteins, glycoproteins (antigens), cell-mediated (non-IgE), or mixed IgE/cell-mediated [27] • Allergies caused by foods affect 1%–10% of the global population, and it is known that approximately 90% of food allergies worldwide are caused by eight major allergens: eggs, milk, crustaceans, shellfish, fish, peanuts, nuts, soybeans, and wheat, which must be clearly identified on product labels by food manufacturers [29]

are based on detection potential or current originated from redox processes at the sensing surface. As the antibodies or nucleic acid aptamers alone are electrically inactive, the redox labels, enzyme labels, or redox mediators are required for application of electrochemical methods [24]. Additionally, nucleic acid aptamers represent a good alternative to the antibodies. These aptamers are characterized by similar specificity to the targets like antibodies. However, aptamers are more flexible, stable, and cheaper in comparison with antibodies. Single-strain DNA sequences are also used as receptors in biosensors hybridizing to specific gene sequences of pathogens, requiring in this case a previous step of extraction of microorganism DNA to be detected [8].

As described by authors of several articles, bioreceptors are immobilized and orientated on the transducer composed of electrodes with different sensing designs. Gold nanoparticles (AuNPs) are often used in electrochemical biosensors due to their excellent electrical properties, label electroactivity, good biocompatibility, easy functionalization, and low signal-to-noise ratio [24,30]. Graphene oxide (GO) and carbon nanotubes have strong electrical conductivity and a large specific surface area, which can accelerate the transfer of electrons and fix more bioreceptors on electrode surfaces [23,31]. The diversity of electrochemical biosensors with different sensing designs is great and some of those already reported in the literature are gold SPEs [30]; Au/Cr interdigitated electrodes [32]; graphene−graphene oxide layer embedded on commercial screen-printed carbon electrodes [33]; graphene surface with AuNPs [31]; reduced graphene oxide-poly(vinyl alcohol), and AuNP nanocomposite (AuNPs/rGO-PVA/GCE) [34]; AuNPs embedded on commercial screen-printed carbon electrodes [35]; carbon paste electrode (CPE) modified with single-walled carbon nanotubes (SWCNTs) onto a printed paper substrate; Pt/Ir electrodes modified with reduced graphene oxide and nanoplatinum [36]; pencil graphite electrode with chitosan/pyrrole (Chi-Py) on multiwalled carbon nanotubes (MWCNTs) and AuNPs [22]; screen-printed carbon electrodes with a composite nanomaterial of graphene oxide−chitosan (GO−CS), and cerium oxide−chitosan (CeO_2−CS) [23]; screen-printed carbon electrode modified with AuNPs and nanoparticles of a polypyrrole (PPy)-electrochemically reduced graphene oxide (ErGO) [37]; indium tin oxide (ITO)-coated glass electrode modified with graphitic carbon nitride (g-C_3N_4) [38].

Independent of associating with nanomaterials or not, there is a consensus that the most sensitive electrochemical detection system used in electrochemical immunosensors and electrochemical aptasensors involves the techniques of EIS, amperometry, and voltammetry. EIS-based biosensors are now among the most commonly used platforms for pathogen detection with minimum sample preparation [8,39]. These techniques coupled with sensing strategies present analytical figures of merit with good results on detection of pathogens in food (milk, chicken, egg, vegetables, and apple juice): linear range of 10^1-10^9 (CFU/mL); limit of detection of 1−67 (CFU/mL); assay time of 20−240 minutes [26].

Besides food contamination by pathogens, the widespread use of pesticides has raised major global health concerns due to their tendency to persist in the environment due to bioaccumulation and potentially contaminate foods. Considering the severe health threats posed by pesticides (infertility, nervous system disorders, immunological, and resultant tract diseases in humans and animals), many efforts have been undertaken to limit their human exposure by restricting the use of pesticides and lowering the limits of maximum residue levels in various matrices and food commodities [40]. Electrochemical sensors, due to their advantages such as sensitivity and selectivity have also been applied in the detection of pesticides providing an approach more eco-friendly, cheaper, and faster than most conventional methods as gas chromatography mass spectrometry (GC−MS) and HPLC−MS [40,41]. Different materials such as metals, metal oxides, conductive polymers, and carbon allotropes such as graphene, fullerene, and SWCNTs or MWCNTs have been used in pesticide electrochemical sensors [9,42]. Nonenzymatic-electrochemical sensors based on carbon allotropes modified with ferrocene−thiophene [43], polypyrrole [44], molybdenum disulfide (MoS_2) [45], $Nd_2Mo_3O_9$ [46], gadolinium oxide (Gd_2O_3) [47], nickel oxide nanoparticles (NiO NPs) [48], pralidoxime (PAM) [49], niobium carbide@molybdenum (NbC@Mo) [50], and others are nanocomposite materials used to increase the surface area, electroactivity, conductivity, and selectivity of the sensors. The synergistic effect obtained with such substrates has generated promising results for the detection of several pesticides such as parathion, chlorantraniliprole, chlorpyrifos, fenthion, endosulfan, carbendazim, and glyphosate pesticides with low LoDs, wide linear measurement range, and almost no interference with other pesticides. Electrochemical biosensors containing antibodies, aptamers, molecularly imprinted polymers (MIPs), and enzyme bioreceptors are other sensing platforms for pesticides have been well reported in scientific literature by many publications and reviews [41,51−54].

Despite the recent progress on electrochemical (bio)sensors, they still lack the ability to identify different contaminants in complex matrices as food samples. Different contaminants influence the electron transfer on the electrode surface, affecting the sensitivity and precision of an electrochemical (bio)sensor. Recently, the developments in computer science and statistics have remarkably improved the selectivity of electrochemical sensors toward the quantification of multiple contaminants. ML is a field of artificial intelligence (AI) that selects appropriate algorithms to build a reasonable statistical model from sample data (training data) and establish predictions toward new data (validation data) [1]. The association of electrochemical (bio)sensors with ML can provide the possibility to realize multiquantification of analytes simply by building a regression model that involves the relationship between current–impedance signals and toxicant concentration [55]. In this context, multivariate data analysis and pattern recognition techniques are important tools to conduct the electrochemical (bio)sensor data treatment. Important pattern recognition methods based on unsupervised and supervised learning techniques applied to food safety are described in the next sections.

7.3 Machine learning techniques used in food science and technology

In general, uncertainty is a very relevant aspect in food production, which is a complex process that may show discrepancies between the planned production and the outcome. These differences usually result in environmental impacts as well as economic costs for the company and finally consumers [56,57]. By applying ML, AI-based systems used in food industries are able to identify several issues or even potential problems often even more efficiently than human-based systems. Recently, the use of AI in this area has been increasing to the point where the great majority of food processing industries are now actively using AI to increase precision in their systems and advance the food chain management of demand and supply, predictive analysis, and meticulous logistics [57].

There is a great variety of ML applications in the food industry [57]. ML algorithms are usually divided into four categories: supervised learning, semisupervised learning, unsupervised learning, and reinforcement learning [58], as shown in Fig. 7.4.

1. In supervised learning, the desired outputs for the samples of training sets are known. This is a type of ML that uses labeled training data to learn new models. This labeled data helps the model in making classifications or even predictions about future data [59]. The most common tasks performed in supervised learning are: classification and regression [58]. Classification methods are highly used in the food industry for

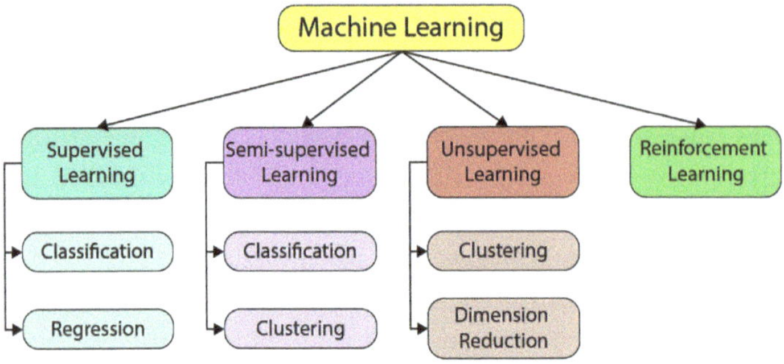

Figure 7.4 Common machine learning categories.

classifying products on the basis of type, quality, and appearance, like detecting misshapen potatoes, assessing the quality of a batch of onions [60], and identifying defective crops [57]. Regression methods are also used in a great variety of applications, such as making predictions for particular systems [61], which is extremely useful for forecasting environmental effects on crop yield, such as weather changes, or for some industry predicting the supply and the demands of its customers [57].

2. Unsupervised learning is widely used as a data-driven approach to find structures, knowledge, or patterns in unlabeled data without the need for human interference [61]. Clustering, dimensionality reduction, density estimation, feature learning, association, and anomaly detection are some of the most common unsupervised learning methods [58]. Clustering is a method that divides the data into several categories according to this data's characteristics [60], then it is commonly used to uncover interesting trends or patterns in data, for example, detect groups of customers according to their behavior [58]. Association rules are used to find relationships between elements in a set of data. Thus, they can be used to estimate the frequency with which a set of items are bought together in a supermarket, and finally, this information is used to improve the user experience when browsing for items [62].
3. Semisupervised learning is a type of ML method that combines labeled and unlabeled data in order to generate a suitable model for classification. In most real-life situations, unlabeled data is abundant, while labeled data could be very difficult to obtain. Therefore, semisupervised classification aims to learn a model that predicts classes of future test data better than that from the model generated using labeled data alone [63].

4. Reinforcement learning is focused on learning by interacting with the environment, taking actions that would maximize the reward or minimize the penalty inside a certain context [63]. This ML method enables the software to automatically reach the best possible behavior for specific circumstances, improving its efficiency. Reinforcement is an extremely valuable type of ML for training AI models that can assist in improving efficiency of operational systems like supply chain logistics or autonomous tasks in general, performed by machines [58].

7.4 Machine learning algorithms applied to food safety and quality inspection

Some of the most important roles of AI in the food industry can be generally divided into two classes: food security management and food quality management [57]. Food safety in this context means ensuring that the food meets the proper nutritional requirements and that it does not contain any potentially toxic substances. Implementing food safety efficiently requires ensuring good hygiene through the production system, which includes food processing, storage, and sale, aiming at reducing the risk of contaminants that could lead to food poisoning. Food quality means that the product needs to meet certain standards in order to be presented to the consumer. This implies that the general aspects of the food, such as appearance, texture, smell, and its components, must be within those standards [60].

As many traditional methods for testing food quality have been considered destructive and not very efficient, many reliable, fast, and nondestructive techniques have been developed over the years for the evaluation of the quality parameters of food products [59]. Those techniques usually include the use of sensors to acquire the necessary information about the internal and external constituents, components, condition, and any other data that may be used to assess the quality and safety of the product [56,58,60].

Statistics is one of the most important theoretical foundations of traditional ML methods. The principal analysis is mainly formed by pattern classification, probability density estimation, regression analysis, and others. Therefore, some related algorithms include decision tree (DT), support vector machine (SVM), Bayesian network (BN), K-nearest neighbors, K-means, fuzzy C-means, and logistic regression [60]. Types of artificial neural networks (ANNs) are also very frequently used in ML to analyze unstructured data, with convolutional neural networks (CNNs) and recurrent neural networks (RNNs) being the most commonly used examples of such [64].

1. DT has a tree-like structure and is composed of internal nodes, leaf nodes, and branches [64]. An example of a DT logic is illustrated in Fig. 7.5, where each internal node represents a decision over a feature, each branch represents the decision output, and each leaf node represents a classification result [60]. Classification and regression tree (CART) and random forest (RF) are some DT models that show great potential and advantages in pattern recognition. CART is described as a single tree with many branches where the dataset is divided following the selected decision. On the other hand, RF is shown as a set of different trees combined using different sets of input variables, which are randomly selected [65].
1. BN, according to Friedman et al. [66], are directed acyclic graphs that allow efficient and effective representation of the joint probability distribution over a set of random variables. Mathematically, with I representing the set of all the nodes in the graph and E representing the set of directed connected line segments, G = (I,E) represents the acyclic graph. With X = (X_i), i ∈ I being a random variable represented by a node i in the graph, X is a BN relative to the directed acyclic graph G (where f(i) are the parents of node i) if the joint probability of the node X can be shown as [60]:

$$p(x) = \prod_{i \in I} p\left(x(i) \middle| x_{\{f(i)\}}\right) \tag{7.1}$$

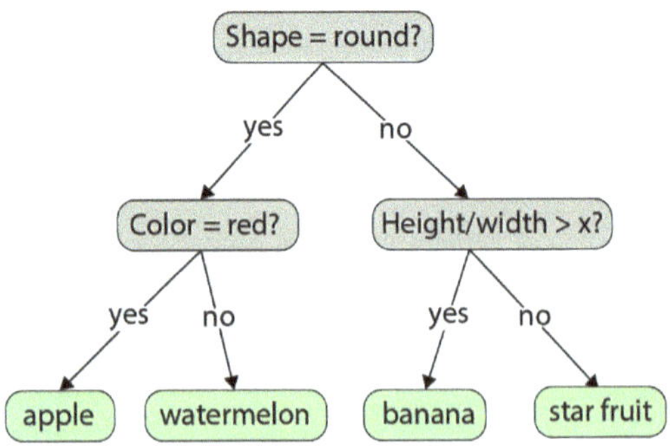

Figure 7.5 Illustration of the logic of a decision tree.

Furthermore, by multiplying those respective local conditional probability distributions, as shown in Eq. (7.2), the joint probability can be obtained for any random variable [60].

$$p(x_1, \ldots, x_n) = p(x_n | x_1, \ldots, x_{n-1}) \ldots p(x_2 | x_1)\, p(x_1) \tag{7.2}$$

1. K-nearest neighbors is an algorithm composed of two parameters that must be set or adjusted and that can, in return, directly affect the classification outcomes. The first parameter, K, is the number of neighbors, while the second one depends on the intended outcome. If regression is intended, the output is the mean of the K labels from the K nearest neighbors. On the other hand, if classification is intended, the output is the simple majority vote of those K nearest neighbors of each point [58,67].
2. K-means is a clustering algorithm and is one of the most used unsupervised ML methods for classifying unlabeled data into groups and for determining cluster centers [67,68]. By choosing the desired number of clusters, the k-means procedure repeatedly moves the centers to minimize the total variance within the cluster. More specifically, it assigns the data points to the K clusters in a way that the average difference between the data points and the cluster mean within each cluster is minimized [68].
3. Fuzzy C-means is one of the most famous soft clustering methods, also known as soft K-means, introduced as an extension of the K-means method [69,70]. It is an unsupervised clustering algorithm applied in various fields including agricultural engineering, chemistry, image analysis, target recognition, and shape analysis in a wide scope of problems related to feature analysis, clustering, and classifier design. The main difference between fuzzy C-means and K-means clustering is that in the former, each data point has a weight associated with every cluster. This works in a way that the closer the data point is to a cluster, the higher is its degree of belonging to this cluster, while a data point that lies farther from the center of the same cluster will present a lower degree of belonging [70].
4. SVM-based ML methods have been largely applied in classification of food products, agricultural crops, detection of adulteration, diseases, seed viability, quantification of chemical components in agricultural elements, and others. SVM approaches focus on acquiring the optimal hyperplanes (which in this case is a vector or a plane that best divides the labeled data in its classes) by selecting those that pass through the

largest possible gaps between points of different classes. The new data points are then allocated to a certain class depending on which side of the surfaces they fall on [59].

5. Logistic regression is an ML algorithm that is widely used for binary classification. In this method, the dependent variable has only two categories, generally represented by 1 (which can represent the occurrence of an event, presence of an element) and 0 (which can stand for absence or failure in a specific context). This model predicts the probability of a target variable with the output being only the two possible classes [71,72].
6. ANN is a structure developed to mimic the functioning of a human brain using as a base the working principle of a biological neuron. The most basic structure of an ANN is a multilayer perceptron, which is made of an input layer, hidden layers, and an output layer. This network is an aggregation of perceptrons with thresholds, weights, and activation function [64]. In a classification context, since the output of an ANN is a nonlinear function of the inputs, the decision boundary can also be nonlinear, making this model more flexible as compared to logistic regression [71] (Fig. 7.6).
7. CNN is a type of deep learning architecture used for feature extraction, and it is generally composed of inputs, convolutional layers,

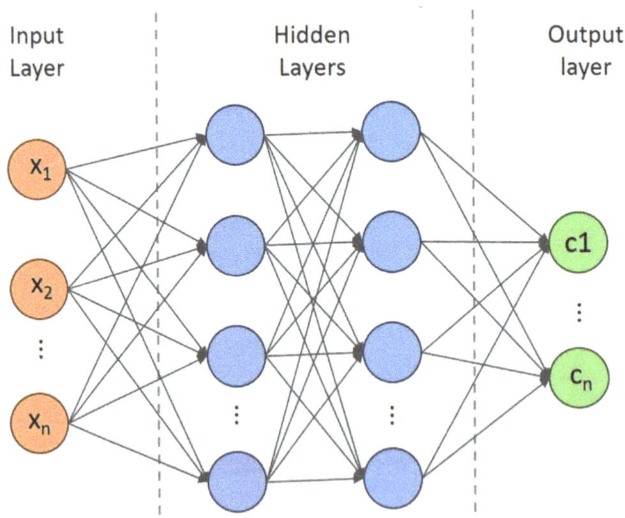

Figure 7.6 Representation of the structure of an artificial neural network with multiple processing layers.

grouping, pooling, fully connected, and dense layers [73]. It is a highly parallelized method based on forward and backward propagation principles, and it can automatically learn to extract features distributed to the input data using convolutional layers. This ML method is widely used for image classification and has been widely studied and used for extracting food features [65].

7.5 Machine learning applied to electrochemical sensors for monitoring food contaminants

The challenges listed for the use of electrochemical sensors are attributed to the lack of signal reproducibility when analyzing real samples and the occurrence of interferences. With the aim to improve the reproducibility and to obtain sensitivity differences in the electroanalytical detection of food contaminants, future approaches require detailed observation of the physical and electrochemical processes at the electrode—electrolyte interface. Besides the use of single peak currents and peak potentials information, there are other important data discarded or neglected during the data analysis procedure. This means that one-dimensional data analysis is typically not enough to acquire sensitive signals highly correlated with the analyte type and quantity [10]. In order to develop an accurate electrochemical screening for the analyte characterization, it is necessary to integrate chemometrics and ML methods [74].

ML as an advanced AI-based data analysis tool can highly improve the field of quantitative voltammetry and can describe even complex electrochemical reactions [75]. Modern and user-friendly computing languages and algorithms can provide methods for quantitative comparison of experimental data with simulated datasets derived from models. Parameters present in the simulated model are related to electrode and chemical kinetics, thermodynamics, mass transport, uncompensated resistance, double-layer capacitance, and electrode area. The principles used to describe these parameters are based on Fick's laws of diffusion for the analysis of mass transport, Ohm's law for modeling uncompensated resistance effects, and the Butler—Volmer and Marcus—Hush theories for the study of heterogeneous electron transfer processes. Despite the potential of ML in quantitative voltammetry, its applications in extracting thermodynamic, kinetic, mass transport, and mechanistic information are scarce to date [75].

The literature concerning electrochemical (bio)sensors coupled with ML for food safety shows that the use of ML methods in current electrochemical (bio)sensors is still in the incipient stages. The works using ML algorithms to analyze sensing data of food contaminants are mainly related to food pathogens, some hazardous toxicants, and in almost all cases, involve the use of EIS technique. EIS has been among the most commonly used platforms for pathogen detection with minimum sample preparation. Changes in the EIS sensors due to pathogenic bacteria are generally reported via the charge transfer resistance (Rct). The sensors are first incubated in the sample to allow the formation of microbial biofilm on the surface, and raw impedance data is measured afterward in a buffer solution with an added redox-active moiety. Thus, a linear relationship can be established between the Rct and bacterial concentration. To potentially improve the EIS sensory performance, an alternative could be to perform multiparameter analysis integrating more impedimetric parameters such as ohmic resistance of the solution or double-layer capacitance to report system changes induced by pathogens [76]. Since more dimensions of EIS data are explored, the accuracy in bacterial detection could be improved.

ML is superior for solving multiparameter and nonlinear problems, due to its self-learning ability [76]. Xu et al. [76] improved accuracy in determining *E. coli* concentration when establishing a quantitative relationship between multiple impedimetric parameters and *E. coli* concentrations. The authors used both capacitance and resistance information to formulate an ML model by using principal component analysis (PCA) and support vector regression (SVR). In another study, Ying Xu et al. [77] proposed an ML-based EIS biosensor method to detect the effect of a low-dose inhibitor (e.g., hydrogen peroxide) on *E. coli*. The target bacteria EIS was immobilized to the electrode surface (multiwalled carbon nanotube-Prussian blue-gold nanoparticle (MWCNT-PB-AuNPs) through antibodies data, and the impedance parameters were obtained. XGBoost and SVR ML models were compared to establish a quantitative relationship between multiple impedance parameters (Cdl-T: interfacial capacitance of the electrode solution, Rs: the resistance of the solution, and Rp: polarization resistance) and the bacterial concentration under the effect of growth inhibitors. The maximum prediction error of the inhibitor concentration training by XGBoost was 4.95%.

The study by Hatorri et al. [78] brought a very interesting methodological approach to identify five different bacteria (*S. aureus*, *Pseudomonas fluorescens*,

S. enterica, *E. coli*, and *Bacillus cereus*) using an electrochemical sensor associated with ML. The sensor was built based on the Coulter principle, which says that particles or cells in a fluid attracted to a microchannel cause a brief change in the electrical resistance of the liquid. The associated transient change in the ionic current (I_{ion}) through the pore was measured using a pair of Ag—AgCl electrodes under the applied voltage. Classification of eight resistive pulse patterns (including height; width; pulse peak position; area, and others) were defined and exploited in an ML-based classification of resistive pulses (Weka workbench with rotation forest ensembles). From the output of the algorithm on each labeled signal, the rates of true-negative, true-positive, false-negative, and false-positive cases were estimated. The model resulted in a 91% accuracy for identifying the bacteria from the I_{ion} signature profiles at a single-cell level. The well-presented technique is very rapid and may be used for real-time screening of pathogenic bacteria for food, environmental, and medical applications.

Aiming to offer low cost and disposable biosensors for food pathogens detection available everywhere in developing countries, the building of dispositives as reported by Ali et al. [79] become very useful. The authors proposed a novel impedance-based biosensor that could detect three different types of bacteria, including *E. coli* strains JM 109 and DH5-α, and *Salmonella typhimurium* with data treatment performed by using various ML algorithms to classify them. The optimized biosensor loaded into the probe station was based on silver interdigital electrodes with 200 μm fingers spacing and decorated with an Ag nanowire concentration of $30 \times 10^3/mm^2$ on a polyethylene terephthalate substrate. The difference among the impedance of the three species of bacteria had a small value, which was difficult to detect with a conventional ohmmeter. To make a reliable classification of pathogens, the algorithms maximum likelihood, linear discriminant analysis, and back-propagation artificial neural network were used. The classification involved the voltage sweeping applied of ±2.5 V with 251 steps and the resulting current (I) values. The sample impedance was measured from the voltage and current values for the voltage sweep of ±2.5 V. The ML algorithms exhibited a good performance and clearly separated each bacteria type by classifying 100%.

Another analytical approach employed in food safety issues is the electronic nose (E-nose), which is a possible alternative method in the identification and classification of different chemicals and bacteria. Their sensing platform can analyze volatile organic compounds produced by microorganisms in a rapid and noninvasive online monitoring approach. These volatiles provide fingerprints for microorganisms and can be employed for pathogen identification and discrimination without the use of conventional food analysis techniques [80]. The application of E-nose for pathogen detection is described in detail in several articles [79,81]. Metal oxide semiconductors (MOS) have been commonly used as sensing elements in E-nose devices due to their availability, high sensitivity, and the ability to respond to the compound's electroactivity. The gas molecules adsorbed on the MOS sensor cause change in conductivity. Polymers (polypyrroles, thiophenes, indoles polyaniline) also have been used as sensing elements. The main components of an E-nose device are: (1) a chemical sensor array; (2) a pattern recognition system equipped with a signal processing mechanism; and (3) an odor sample collector [79]. The E-nose pattern recognition system is based on ML algorithms employed for prediction of possible food mycotoxins and pathogens. Pattern recognition algorithms used are: PCA, discriminant analysis (DA), partial least squares, discriminant function analysis (DFA), ANN, and SVM. The classification accuracy obtained from the pattern recognition tool can achieve a range of 80%−100% accuracy [80]. The overall effectiveness of the pattern recognition algorithm applied is ensured by extracting robust information from sensor responses with less redundancy. Pattern recognition methods for E-nose are described in the review article of [80,81]. E-nose technique offers advantages in food application as it has remarkable potential in the practical routine analysis compared to other inspection methods such as the lack of sample preparations, with no need to use organic solvents, and to conduct derivatization, which is widely used in chemical analyses. The disadvantages and challenges of E-nose technique are related to: (1) requirement for odor discrimination or differentiation data training usually performed by correlating E-nose responses with chromatography (GC, HPLC); (2) inability to recognize individual chemical compounds within the gas odors together with the adverse implications of humidity and temperature [79]; (3) less reliability of output signal of the array sensor due to the cross-interference caused by irrelevant gasses [79].

The association of ML methods and electrochemical biosensors applied to the determination of nonbiological food contaminants provided the very first possibility to realize the quantification of multiple toxicants by regressing a model of the internal relationship between current signals and toxicant information [55]. Many sensing platforms are useful to detect water pollutants but can be also used as promising tools for food safety purposes. Massah and Vakilian [81] developed an intelligent portable biosensor by using an enzyme-based three-electrode electrochemical unit to determine nitrate concentration in beverages and water. SVM learning with polynomial kernel function method was used to predict the nitrate concentration considering the electrocatalytic response of the sample obtained by cyclic voltammetry using a glassy carbon/enzyme electrode. The sensing platform was connected to an iPhone through Bluetooth for decision-making and displaying the results. Results showed that the trained algorithm resulted in promising nitrate prediction accuracy with values of R^2 and mean squared error of 0.93 and 0.0016, respectively. The great advantages offered by the method were: simple operation; biosensor lifetime at least 10 days; analytical capacity of 400 samples in 10 days without the need for enzyme replacement; nitrate working range concentrations from 0 to 2000 mM; the nitrate concentration measured by the proposed system is very similar to the values measured by spectrophotometric method; possibility to share the results though a mobile application on an iPhone wirelessly connected to the device.

Xu et al. [82] designed a low-cost disposable electrochemical sensing platform for analysis of maleic hydrazide (MH) in food. The electrochemical measurements were performed by a conventional three-electrode system, which consisted of a disposable laser-induced porous graphene electrode, a saturated calomel electrode (SCE), and a platinum electrode that served as the working electrode, reference electrode, and counter electrode. Differential pulse voltammetry was carried to the MH current voltages measurements. Different algorithms such as ANN, RF, and least squares support vector machine (LS-SVM) were selected to build the ML models. The input data was the current values measured by MH, and the output data was its predicted concentration values. In comparison with the performance of the models, LS-SVM was more able to predict the concentration of MH in the range of 0.9–101.9 μM (training: R^2 (coefficient of determination) = 0.9999; RMSEC (root mean square error of calibration) = 0.3880/ prediction: $R^2 = 0.9994$; RMSEP (root mean square error of prediction) = 0.7717). After satisfactory recoveries of MH in potato and peanuts (99.07%–104.80%, with RSD range of 1.12%–1.56%), the LS-SVM model was proved to be feasible and reliable for practical prediction in analyzing MH in real samples.

Heavy metals and pesticides are considered potential inorganic hazardous chemicals to the environment and food and can be detected by voltammetry with high sensitivity. The reproducibility and selectivity of electroanalytical sensors can be highly improved to detect these contaminants by chemometrics and ML by developing fingerprint electroanalytical approaches for the identification of food contaminants. A bacterial biosensor array (or multisensor) was fabricated by immobilizing three types of bacterial cells on the surface of screen-printed gold electrodes via poly L-lysine (PLl) to detect heavy metals, pesticides, and hydrocarbons (Hg(II), Pb(II), Cd(II), atrazine, simazine, hexane, pentane, pyrene, toluene, octane, and ethanol) in water [83]. Electrochemical measurements by cyclic voltammetry and impedance spectra were carried out on electrodes coated with immobilized bacteria, in buffer solutions containing different pollutant concentrations. The bacteria (*E. coli*, *Methylococcus capsulatus*, and *Shewanella oneidensis*) immobilized on the electrodes acted as insulators reducing the charge transfer at the electrode surface. However, bacteria are damaged by exposure to pollutants, and their insulating properties are reduced. The comparison of the effect of different concentrations of pollutants on the bacteria was performed by a normalized input dataset of CV measurements of anodic current at +0.5 V. The inhibition effect of 12 pollutants studied lied in the reduction of bacterial electrical resistivity. The accurate recognition of pollutants was achieved with the use of ANN considering three layers: (1) the different bacteria; (2) 12 neurons corresponding to 12 pollutants studied; and (3) the output layer representing a six-digit binary code, which identifies the type of pollutants and their concentration.

Ye et al. [74] combined PCA with SVM to classify the electroanalytical signals of six heavy metals (Cu(II), Cd(II), Hg(II), Pb(II), Zn(II), and Ag(I)) based on their voltammetric peak shapes using bare-glassy carbon electrode, where the absolute values of the current and potential were not under consideration. The authors assumed that the voltammetric peak shape, which is a potential-dependent reaction, minimizes error due reliance on the reference electrode and the active surface area of the working electrode. To train the dataset, 140 square-wave voltammetry (SWV) experiments for the six heavy metal ions (HMIs) were used, while another 60 SWV experiments were used as the testing data set. For the SWV peak, the first to sixth principal components covered 99% of the overall variance for the 140 training samples. The SVM classifier identified the SWV signal from Cu, Hg, Zn, and Ag with 100% accuracy. For Cd and Pb, which exhibit similar current responses, most signals could be correctly identified with an accuracy of 90%. Without the assistance of the

ML classifier, it was impossible to distinguish the SWV peak shapes of Cd (II) and Pb(II).

In a recent study, Du et al. [55] built a microbial electrochemical sensor to detect and quantify $MnCl_2$, $NaNO_2$, and tetracycline hydrochloride (TCH) in water. Electrochemical activity of a biofilm and toxicity were extracted from chronoamperometry (current − time) measurements before and after the injection of toxicants. By using regression ML models with different algorithms (SVM, ANN, and a generalized linear model), a functional relationship between electrochemical data (input) and concentrations of toxicants (output) as training set was generated. Based on the model, the concentration prediction of each type of toxicant was calculated with satisfactory accuracy.

7.6 Conclusions and perspectives

The growing world demand for food and future forecasts strengthen the need to maintain and develop more and more safe and quality food for society. The adoption of fast, lower-cost, sensitive, selective, and available analytical techniques at all stages of food processing will be extremely necessary in the context of food safety and quality. This chapter has described the main types of electrochemical (bio)sensors applied to the analysis of food contaminants, their main innovations for better sensing performance, and the use of ML for data processing and prediction. Electrochemical (bio)sensors offer several advantages in comparison with conventional methods as they are very sensitive, have good selectivity, excellent repeatability, and accuracy, and are less expensive than most other high-performance detection tools. The successful integration of nanomaterial-based interfaces and novel sensing platforms with biorecognition tools (antibodies, aptamers, and imprinted polymers) have improved electrochemical sensors for the ultra-trace quantification and identification of several contaminants (biological and nonbiological). Other analytical advantages include a faster analysis with simplified analytical processes and the possibility of miniaturization and portability. In contrast, electrochemical sensors offer some disadvantages such as short/limited life; limited ability to detect more than one pathogenic contaminant (multiplexing detection); no widespread commercialization and using on-site or in industrial food control applications; and currently represent good alternatives to conventional methods of analysis in laboratory scale. To face these challenges, efforts are necessary: to improve the construction of synthetic receptors (such as MIPs and aptamers) fixed on nanomaterials interfaces; to enhance the analytical efficiency of electrochemical (bio)sensors by complete validation of biosensors and application to real samples with minimal pretreatment; to facilitate the commercialization of electrochemical (bio)sensors by making progress of on-site methods of analysis using lab-on-a-chip tools at low cost and smartphones as portable interfaces.

The perspectives about developing arrayed or multiplexing electrochemical bio(sensors) able to test numerous real samples opened opportunities for the application of deep learning in electrochemical (bio)sensors. The combination of electrochemical sensing and ML could quantitatively improve the molecular recognition ability and optimize the experimental parameters of the electrical biosensor device. ML brought new opportunities to the electrochemical sensing widespread utilization extracting features and predicting the species and concentration of the analytes. The use of ML for food safety and food quality monitoring and prediction is still considerably recent, but one that is also rapidly increasing due to its promising results. With the growing technology devoted to sensors, their applications in the food industry likewise increase and expand, and with that, more ML methods are used in ever-wider ranges of applications, from data processing, classification, prediction, to improving sensor reliability. In ML, each algorithm is developed, adapted, or modified for specific purposes and, as this area continues to exponentially grow, more studies are performed aiming to obtain more efficient results for different kinds of data. Hence, using the right model for specific data results in higher accuracies and more efficient systems.

References

[1] A.M. Jiménez-Carvelo, A. González-Casado, M. Gracia Bagur-González, L. Cuadros-Rodríguez, Alternative data mining/machine learning methods for the analytical evaluation of food quality and authenticity — a review, Food Res. Int. 122 (2019) 25—39. Available from: https://doi.org/10.1016/j.foodres.2019.03.063.

[2] A.G.-M. Ferrari, R.D. Crapnell, C.E. Banks, Electroanalytical overview: electrochemical sensing platforms for food and drink safety, Biosensors 11 (2021) 291. Available from: https://doi.org/10.3390/bios11080291.

[3] M.A. Shenashen, M.Y. Emran, A.E. Sabagh, M.M. Selim, A. Elmarakbi, S.A. El-Safty, Progress in sensory devices of pesticides, pathogens, coronavirus, and chemical additives and hazards in food assessment: food safety concerns, Prog. Mater. Sci. 124 (2022) 100866. Available from: https://doi.org/10.1016/j.pmatsci.2021.100866.

[4] FAO and WHO, Codex Alimentarius Commission – Procedural Manual, 27th ed., FAO and WHO, Rome, 2019. Available from: https://www.fao.org/3/ca2329en/ca2329en.pdf. (accessed 20.09.22).
[5] R.S. Rodriguez, T.L. O'Keefe, C. Froehlich, R.E. Lewis, et al., Sensing food contaminants: advances in analytical methods and techniques, Anal. Chem. 93 (2021) 23–40. Available from: https://doi.org/10.1021/acs.analchem.0c04357.
[6] G. Bülbül, A. Hayat, S. Andreescu, Portable nanoparticle-based sensors for food safety assessment, Sensors 15 (2015) 30736–30758. Available from: https://doi.org/10.3390/s151229826.
[7] G.K. Mishra, A. Barfidokht, F. Tehrani, R.K. Mishra, Food safety analysis using electrochemical biosensors, Foods 7 (2018) 141. Available from: https://doi.org/10.3390/foods7090141.
[8] M. Amiri, A. Bezaatpour, H. Jafari, R. Boukherroub, S. Szunerits, Electrochemical methodologies for the detection of pathogens, ACS Sens. 3 (2018) 1069–1086. Available from: https://doi.org/10.1021/acssensors.8b00239.
[9] Y. Li, Z. Wang, L. Sun, L. Liu, C. Xu, H. Kuang, Nanoparticle-based sensors for food contaminants, Trends Anal. Chem. 113 (2019) 74–83. Available from: https://doi.org/10.1016/j.trac.2019.01.012.
[10] F. Cui, Y. Yue, Y. Zhang, Z. Zhang, H. Susan Zhou, Advancing biosensors with machine learning, ACS Sens. 5 (2020) 3346–3364. Available from: https://doi.org/10.1021/acssensors.0c01424.
[11] S. Namuduri, B.N. Narayanan, V. Salini, P. Davuluru, et al., Review—deep learning methods for sensor based predictive maintenance and future perspectives for electrochemical sensors, J. Electrochem. Soc. 167 (2020) 037552. Available from: https://doi.org/10.1149/1945-7111/ab67a8.
[12] A. Singh, A. Sharma, A. Ahmed, A.K. Sundramoorthy, H. Furukawa, S. Arya, et al., Recent advances in electrochemical biosensors: applications, challenges, and future scope, Biosensors 11 (2021) 336. Available from: https://doi.org/10.3390/bios11090336.
[13] J. Wang, Analytical Electrochemistry, Second ed., Wiley-VCH, New York, 2000.
[14] V.S. Manikandan, B. Adhikarib, A. Chen, Nanomaterial based electrochemical sensors for the safety and quality control of food and beverages, Analyst 143 (2018) 4537–4554. Available from: https://doi.org/10.1039/c8an00497h.
[15] D.A. Skoog, F.J. Holler, Te.A. Nieman, Pricípios de Análise Instrumental, 5ª ed., Bookman, Porto Alegre, 2006, p. 836.
[16] J. Bunney, S. Williamson, D. Atkin, M. Jeanneret, D. Cozzolino, J. Chapman, et al., The use of electrochemical biosensors in food analysis, Curr. Res. Nutr. Food Sci. 5 (3) (2017) 183–195. Available from: https://doi.org/10.12944/CRNFSJ.5.3.02.
[17] E. Jubete, O.A. Loaiza, E. Ochoteco, J.A. Pomposo, Nanotechnology: a tool for improved performance on electrochemical screen-printed (bio)sensors, Hindawi Publ. Corporation J. Sens. (2009) 13. Available from: https://doi.org/10.1155/2009/842575. ID 842575.
[18] V. Kumar, P. Guleria, S.K. Mehta, Nanosensors for food quality and safety assessment, Env. Chem. Lett. 15 (2017) 165–177. Available from: https://doi.org/10.1007/s10311-017-0616-4.
[19] S. Raja, M. Vedhanayagam, D.R. Preeth, C. Kim, J.H. Lee, D.W. Han, Development of two dimensional nanomaterials based electrochemical biosensors on enhancing the analysis of food toxicants, Int. J. Mol. Sci. 22 (2021) 3277. Available from: https://doi.org/10.3390/ijms22063277.
[20] A.D. Ambaye, K.K. Kefeni, S.B. Mishra, E.N. Nxumalo, B. Ntsendwana, Recent developments in nanotechnology-based printing electrode systems for electrochemical sensors, Talanta 225 (2021) 121951. Available from: https://doi.org/10.1016/j.talanta.2020.121951.

[21] G. Yunus, M. Kuddus, Electrochemical biosensor for food borne pathogens: an overview, Carpathian J. Food Sci. Technol. 12 (2) (2020) 5–16. Available from: https://doi.org/10.34302/crpjfst/2020.12.2.1.
[22] A. Güner, E. Çevik, M. Senel, L. Alpsoy, An electrochemical immunosensor for sensitive detection of *Escherichia coli* O157:H7 by using chitosan, MWCNT, polypyrrole with gold nanoparticles hybrid sensing platform, Food Chem. 229 (2017) 358–365. Available from: https://doi.org/10.1016/j.foodchem.2017.02.083.
[23] X. An, X. Shi, H. Zhang, Y. Yao, G. Wang, Q. Yang, et al., An electrochemical immunosensor based on a combined amplification strategy with the GO–CS/CeO_2–CS nanocomposite for the detection of aflatoxin M_1, New J. Chem. 44 (2020) 1362–1370. Available from: https://doi.org/10.1039/c9nj04804a.
[24] V. Subjakova, V. Oravczova, M. Tatarko, T. Hianik, Advances in electrochemical aptasensors and immunosensors for detection of bacterial pathogens in food, Electrochim 389 (2021) 138724. Available from: https://doi.org/10.1016/j.electacta.2021.138724.
[25] M. Sundhoro, S.R. Agnihotra, N.D. Khan, A. Barnes, J. BelBruno, L. Mendecki, Rapid and accurate electrochemical sensor for food allergen detection in complex foods, Sci. Rep. 11 (2021) 20831. Available from: https://doi.org/10.1038/s41598-021-00241-6.
[26] J. Riu, B. Giussani, Electrochemical biosensors for the detection of pathogenic bacteria in food, Trends Anal. Chem. 126 (2020) 115863. Available from: https://doi.org/10.1016/j.trac.2020.115863.
[27] J. Zhang, L. Lu, Z. Zhang, L. Zang, Electrochemical cell-based sensor for detection of food hazards, Micromachines 12 (2021) 837. Available from: https://doi.org/10.3390/mi12070837.
[28] S.M. Taghdisi, N.M. Danesh, M. Ramezani, M. Alibolandi, M.A. Nameghi, G. Gerayelou, et al., A novel electrochemical aptasensor for ochratoxin sensing in spiked food using strand-displacement polymerase reaction, Talanta 223 (2021) 121705. Available from: https://doi.org/10.1016/j.talanta.2020.121705.
[29] S. Campuzano, V.R.-V. Montiel, V. Serafín, P. Yáñez-Sedeño, J.M. Pingarrón, Cutting-edge advances in electrochemical affinity biosensing at different molecular level of emerging food allergens and adulterants, Biosensors 10 (2020) 10. Available from: https://doi.org/10.3390/bios10020010.
[30] L. Li, M. Zhang, W. Chen, Gold nanoparticle-based colorimetric and electrochemical sensors for the detection of illegal food aditives, J. Food Drug. Anal. 28 (4) (2020). Available from: https://doi.org/10.38212/2224-6614.3114. Article 10.
[31] Y. Guo, Y. Wang, S. Liu, J. Yu, H. Wang, M. Cui, et al., Electrochemical immunosensor assay (EIA) for sensitive detection of *E. coli* O157:H7 with signal amplification on a SG-PEDOT-AuNPs electrode interface, Analyst 140 (2015) 551–559. Available from: https://doi.org/10.1039/c4an01463d.
[32] I. Jasim, Z. Shen, Z. Mlaji, N.S. Yuksek, A. Abdullah, J.S. Liu, et al., An impedance biosensor for simultaneous detection of low concentration of *Salmonella* serogroups in poultry and fresh produce samples, Biosens. Bioelectron. 126 (2019) 292–300. Available from: https://doi.org/10.1016/j.bios.2018.10.065.
[33] R. Mutreja, M. Jariyal, P. Pathania, A. Sharma, D.K. Sahoo, C.R. Suri, Novel surface antigen based impedimetric immunosensor for detection of *Salmonella typhimurium* in water and juice samples, Biosens. Bioelectron. 85 (2016) 707–713. Available from: https://doi.org/10.1016/j.bios.2016.05.079.
[34] M. Qaanei, R.A. Taheri, K. Eskandari, Electrochemical aptasensor for: *Escherichia coli* O157:H7 bacteria detection using a nanocomposite of reduced graphene oxide, gold nanoparticles and polyvinyl alcohol, Anal. Methods 13 (27) (2021) 3101–3109. Available from: https://doi.org/10.1039/d1ay00563d.

[35] X. Mo, Z. Wu, J. Huang, G. Zhao, W. Dou, A sensitive and regenerative electrochemical immunosensor for quantitative detection of: *Escherichia coli* O157:H7 based on stable polyaniline coated screen-printed carbon electrode and rGO-NR-Au@Pt, Anal. Methods 11 (2019) 1475–1482. Available from: https://doi.org/10.1039/c8ay02594k.

[36] K.D. Hills, D.A. Oliveira, N.D. Cavallaro, C.L. Gomes, E.S. McLamore, Actuation of chitosan-aptamer nanobrush borders for pathogen sensing, Analyst 143 (2018) 1650–1661. Available from: https://doi.org/10.1039/c7an02039b.

[37] L. Lu, R. Seenivasan, Y.-C. Wang, J.-H. Yu, S. Gunasekaran, An electrochemical immunosensor for rapid and sensitive detection of mycotoxins fumonisin B1 and deoxynivalenol, Electrochim. Acta 213 (2016) 89–97. Available from: https://doi.org/10.1016/j.electacta.2016.07.096.

[38] V. Nirbhaya, D. Chauhan, R. Jain, R. Chandra, S. Kumar, Nanostructured graphitic carbon nitride based ultrasensing electrochemical biosensor for food toxin detection, Bioelectrochem 139 (2021) 107738. Available from: https://doi.org/10.1016/j.bioelechem.2021.107738.

[39] Z. Farka, T. Juřík, M. Pastucha, D. Kovar, K. Lacina, P. Skladal, Rapid immunosensing of Salmonella typhimurium using electrochemical impedance spectroscopy: the effect of sample treatment, Electroanal 28 (2016) 1803–1809. Available from: https://doi.org/10.1002/elan.201600093.

[40] N. Kaur, A. Khunger, S.L. Wallen, A. Kaushik, G.R. Chaudhary, R.S. Varma, Advanced green analytical chemistry for environmental pesticide detection, Curr. Opin. Green. Sustain. Chem. 30 (2021) 100488. Available from: https://doi.org/10.1016/j.cogsc.2021.100488.

[41] M. Majdinasab, M. Daneshi, J.L. Marty, Recent developments in non-enzymatic (bio)sensors for detection of pesticide residues: focusing on antibody, aptamer and molecularly imprinted polymer, Talanta 232 (2021) 122397. Available from: https://doi.org/10.1016/j.talanta.2021.122397.

[42] M. Bhattu, M. Verma, D. Kathuria, Recent advancements in the detection of organophosphate pesticides: a review, Anal. Methods 13 (2021) 4390. Available from: https://doi.org/10.1039/d1ay01186c.

[43] S.O. Tümay, A. Şenocak, E. Sarı, V. Sanko, M. Durmus, E. Demirbas, A new perspective for electrochemical determination of parathion and chlorantraniliprole pesticides via carbon nanotube-based thiophene-ferrocene appended hybrid nanosensor, Sens. Actuators B Chem. 345 (2021) 130344. Available from: https://doi.org/10.1016/j.snb.2021.130344.

[44] S. Ding, Z. Lyu, S. Li, X. Ruan, M. Fei, Y. Zhou, et al., Molecularly imprinted polypyrrole nanotubes based electrochemical sensor for glyphosate detection, Biosens. Bioelectron. 191 (2021) 113434. Available from: https://doi.org/10.1016/j.bios.2021.113434.

[45] X. Zhu, P. Liu, Y. Ge, R. Wu, T. Xue, Y. Sheng, et al., MoS2/MWCNTs porous nanohybrid network with oxidase-like characteristic as electrochemical nanozyme sensor coupled with machine learning for intelligent analysis of carbendazim, J. Electroanal. Chem. 862 (2020) 113940. Available from: https://doi.org/10.1016/j.jelechem.2020.113940.

[46] Y. Xie, F. Gao, X. Tu, X. Ma, R. Dai, Flake-like neodymium molybdate wrapped with multi-walled carbon nanotubes as an effective electrode material for sensitive electrochemical detection of carbendazim, J. Electroanal. Chem. 855 (2019) 113468. Available from: https://doi.org/10.1016/j.jelechem.2019.113468.

[47] K. Alagumalai, R. Shanmugam, S. Chen, B. Thirumalraj, A.S. Haidyrah, C. Karuppiah, Impact of gadolinium oxide with functionalized carbon nanosphere: a portable advanced electrocatalyst for pesticide detection in aqueous environmental

samples, Talanta 238 (2022) 123028. Available from: https://doi.org/10.1016/j.talanta.2021.
[48] H. Bakhsh, J. Buledi, N.H. Khand, B. Junejo, A.R. Solangi, A. Mallah, et al., NiO nanostructures based functional non-enzymatic electrochemical sensor for ultrasensitive determination of endosulfan in vegetables, J. Food Meas. Charact. 15 (2021) 2695–2704. Available from: https://doi.org/10.1007/s11694-021-00860-7.
[49] J. Dong, J. Hou, J. Jiang, S. Ai, Innovative approach for the electrochemical detection of non-electroactive organophosphorus pesticides using oxime as electroactive probe, Anal. Chim. Acta 885 (2015) 92–97. Available from: https://doi.org/10.1016/j.aca.2015.05.033.
[50] M. Govindasamy, U. Rajaji, S.-M. Chen, S. Kumaravel, T.-W. Chen, F.M.A. Al-Hemaid, et al., Detection of pesticide residues (Fenitrothion) in fruit samples based on niobium carbide@molybdenum nanocomposite: an electrocatalytic approach, Anal. Chim. Acta 1030 (2018) 52–60. Available from: https://doi.org/10.1016/j.aca.2018.05.044.
[51] F. Arduini, S. Cinti, V. Scognamiglio, D. Moscone, Nanomaterials in electrochemical biosensors for pesticide detection: advances and challenges in food analysis, Microchim. Acta 183 (7) (2016) 2063–2083. Available from: https://doi.org/10.1007/s00604-016-1858-8.
[52] X. Zhang, D. Wu, X. Zhou, Y. Yu, J. Liu, N. Hu, et al., Recent progress in the construction of nanozyme-based biosensors and their applications to food safety assay, Trends Anal. Chem. 121 (2019) 115668. Available from: https://doi.org/10.1016/j.trac.2019.115668.
[53] K. Phopin, T. Tantimongcolwat, Pesticide aptasensors—state of the art and perspectives, Sensors (Switz.) 20 (23) (2020) 1–40. Available from: https://doi.org/10.3390/s20236809.
[54] S.S. BaHashwan, M.H.B.M. Khir, Y. Al-Douri, A.Y. Ahmed, Recent progress in the development of biosensors for chemicals and pesticides detection, IEEE Access 8 (2020) 82514–82527. Available from: https://doi.org/10.1109/ACCESS.2020.2991380.
[55] L. Du, Y. Yan, T. Li, H. Liu, N. Li, X. Wang, Machine learning enables quantification of multiple toxicants with microbial electrochemical sensors, ACS EST. Eng. 2 (2022) 92–100. Available from: https://doi.org/10.1021/acsestengg.1c00287.
[56] A. Garre, M.C. Ruiz, E. Hontoria, Application of machine learning to support production planning of a food industry in the context of waste generation under uncertainty, Oper. Res. Perspect. 7 (2020) 100147. Available from: https://doi.org/10.1016/j.orp.2020.100147.
[57] I. Kumar, et al., Opportunities of artificial intelligence and machine learning in the food industry, J. Food Qual. 2021 (2021) 4535567. Available from: https://doi.org/10.1155/2021/4535567. ISSN 0146–9428.
[58] I.H. Sarker, Machine learning: algorithms, real-world applications and research directions, SN Computer Sci. 2 (3) (2021) 160. Available from: https://doi.org/10.1007/s42979-021-00592-x.
[59] D. Saha, A. Manickavasagan, Machine learning techniques for analysis of hyperspectral images to determine quality of food products: a review, Curr. Res. Food Sci. 4 (2021) 28–44. Available from: https://doi.org/10.1016/j.crfs.2021.01.002. ISSN 2665–9271.
[60] L. Zhu, et al., Deep learning and machine vision for food processing: a survey, Curr. Res. Food Sci. 4 (2021) 233–249. Available from: https://doi.org/10.1016/j.crfs.2021.03.009. ISSN 2665–9271.
[61] I.H. Sarker, et al., Cybersecurity data science: an overview from machine learning perspective, J. Big Data 7 (1) (2020) 41. Available from: https://doi.org/10.1186/s40537-020-00318-5. ISSN 2196-1115.

[62] R. Agrawal, T. Imielinski, A. Swami, Mining association rules between sets of items in large databases, ACM SIGMOD Rec. 22 (2) (1993) 207–216. Available from: https://doi.org/10.1145/170036.170072.
[63] M. Mohammed, M.B. Khan, E.B.M. Bashier, Machine Learning: Algorithms and Applications, 1st ed., CRC Press, 2016. Available from: https://doi.org/10.1201/9781315371658.
[64] X. Wang, Y. Bouzembrak, A.O. Lansink, H.J. Fels-Klerx, Application of machine learning to the monitoring and prediction of food safety: a review, Compr. Rev. Food Sci. Food Saf. 21 (1) (2022) 416–434. Available from: https://doi.org/10.1111/1541-4337.12868.
[65] Y. Liu, H. Pu, D.W. Sun, Efficient extraction of deep image features using convolutional neural network (CNN) for applications in detecting and analyzing complex food matrices, Trends Food Sci. Technol. 113 (2021) 193–204. Available from: https://doi.org/10.1016/j.tifs.2021.04.042.
[66] N. Friedman, D. Geiger, M. Goldszmidt, Bayesian network classifiers, Mach. Learn. 29 (1997) 131–163. Available from: https://doi.org/10.1023/A:1007465528199.
[67] P.A. Jaskowiak, R.J.G.B. Campello, Comparing Correlation Coefficients as Dissimilarity Measures for Cancer Classification in Gene Expression Data, Brazilian Symposium on Bioinformatics (BSB 2011). 18 (2011). Available from: 10.1.1.208.993.
[68] Q.-Z. Liao, et al., Statistical prediction of waterflooding performance by k-means clustering and empirical modeling, Pet. Sci. 19 (2022) 1139–1152. Available from: https://doi.org/10.1016/j.petsci.2021.12.032. ISSN 1995–8226.
[69] H. Murfi, N. Rosaline, N. Hariadi, Deep autoencoder-based fuzzy c-means for topic detection, Array 13 (2022) 100124. Available from: https://doi.org/10.1016/j.array.2021.100124. ISSN 2590-0056.
[70] S. Ghosh, S. Kumar, Comparative analysis of K-means and fuzzy C-means algorithms, Int. J. Adv. Comput. Sci. Appl. 4 (4) (2013) 406. Available from: https://doi.org/10.14569/ijacsa.2013.040406.
[71] S. Dreiseitl, L. Ohno-Machado, Logistic regression and artificial neural network classification models: a methodology review, J. Biomed. Inform. 35 (5–6) (2002) 352–359. Available from: https://doi.org/10.1016/s1532-0464(03)00034-0.
[72] A.A.T. Fernandes, D.B. Figueiredo Filho, E.C.D. Rocha, W.D.S. Nascimento, Read this paper if you want to learn logistic regression, Rev. de. Sociologia e Política 28 (74) (2020) 406. Available from: https://doi.org/10.1590/1678-987320287406en.
[73] S.S. Nallan Chakravartula, R. Moscetti, G. Bedini, M. Nardella, R. Massantini, Use of convolutional neural network (CNN) combined with FT-NIR spec-troscopy to predict food adulteration: a case study on coffee, Food Control. 135 (2022) 108816. Available from: https://doi.org/10.1016/j.foodcont.2022.108816.
[74] J.-J. Ye, C.-H. Lina, X.-J. Huang, Analyzing the anodic stripping square wave voltammetry of heavy metal ions via machine learning: information beyond a single voltammetric peak, J. Electroanal. Chem. 872 (2020) 113934. Available from: https://doi.org/10.1016/j.jelechem.2020.113934.
[75] L. Gundry, S.-X. Guo, G. Kennedy, J. Keith, et al., Recent advances and future perspectives for automated parameterisation, Bayesian inference and machine learning in voltammetry, Chem. Commun. 57 (2021) 1855–1870. Available from: https://doi.org/10.1039/D0CC07549C.
[76] Y. Xu, C. Li, Y. Jiang, M. Guo, Y. Yang, Y. Yang, et al., Electrochemical impedance spectroscopic detection of *E. coli* with machine learning, J. Electrochem. Soc. 167 (2020) 047508. Available from: https://doi.org/10.1149/1945-7111/ab732f.
[77] Y. Xu, Y. Jiang, C. Li, Y. Chen, Y. Yang, Integration of an XGBoost model and EIS detection to determine the effect of low inhibitor concentrations on *E. coli*, J.

Electroanal. Chem. 877 (2020) 114534. Available from: https://doi.org/10.1016/j.jelechem.2020.114534.
[78] S. Hattori, R. Sekido, I.W. Leong, et al., Machine learning-driven electronic identifications of single pathogenic bacteria, Sci. Rep. 10 (2020) 15525. Available from: https://doi.org/10.1038/s41598-020-72508-3.
[79] S. Ali, A. Hassan, G. Hassan, C.-H. Eun, et al., Disposable all-printed electronic biosensor for instantaneous detection and classification of pathogens, Sci. Rep. 8 (2018) 5920. Available from: https://doi.org/10.1038/s41598-018-24208-2.
[80] E. Bonah, X. Huang, J.H. Aheto, R. Osae, Application of electronic nose as a non-invasive technique for odor fingerprinting and detection of bacterial foodborne pathogens: a review, J. Food Sci. Technol. 57 (6) (2020) 1977−1990. Available from: https://doi.org/10.1007/s13197-019-04143-4.
[81] J. Massah, K. Asefpour Vakilian, An intelligent portable biosensor for fast and accurate nitrate determination using cyclic voltammetry, Biosyst. Eng. (2018) 1−10. Available from: https://doi.org/10.1016/j.biosystemseng.
[82] L. Xu, R. Wu, X. Zhu, X. Wang, et al., Intelligent analysis of maleic hydrazide using a simple electrochemical sensor coupled with machine learning, Anal. Methods 13 (2021) 4662−4673. Available from: https://doi.org/10.1039/D1AY01261D.
[83] H. Abu-Ali, A. Nabok, T.J. Smith, Electrochemical inhibition bacterial sensor array for detection of water pollutants: artificial neural network (ANN) approach, Anal. Bioanal. Chem. 411 (2019) 7659−7668. Available from: https://doi.org/10.1007/s00216-019-01853-8.

Index

Note: Page numbers followed by "*t*" refer to tables.

G

H

I

Y

Z

FSC
www.fsc.org
MIX
Papier | Fördert gute Waldnutzung
FSC® C083411

Kolibri 360 GmbH
Ferdinand-Jühlke-Straße 7
99095 Erfurt, Deutschland
produktsicherheit@kolibri360.de